The
D'ADAMO
DIET

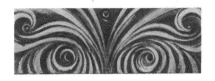

The

D'ADAMO

DIET

A Naturopath tells you how to unlock

the energy, health, and vitality within you

by matching your diet to your blood type.

DR. JAMES D'ADAMO,
Naturopath

HEALTH THRU HERBS
Toronto

1 2 3 4 5 6 7 8 9 10 M 8 7 6 5 4 3 2 1 0 9

Printed and bound in Canada

Canadian Cataloguing in Publication Data
D'Adamo, James,
    The D'Adamo diet

Includes bibliographical references.
ISBN 0-9680232-0-7

1. Diet therapy.   2. Naturopathy.   3. Diet.
4. Blood groups — ABO system.   5. Nutrition.
I. Title.

RM217.D33 1989   615.8'54   C90-093259-7

DESIGN AND COVER ILLUSTRATION: SHARON MATTHEWS
TECHNICAL ILLUSTRATIONS: ANNETTE TATCHELL

*Dedicated to my wife, Christiana
without whose help and
support this book never
could have occurred.*

CONTENTS

INTRODUCTION 1
Why is This Happening to Me? 1
What Can I Do about It? 4

1 COMMITMENT TO HEALTH 5
Results of a Healthy Menu 5
Heal Me, Doctor 7
Is It Really All up to Me? 10
Breaking Food Habits 11

2 BLOOD TYPES 14
Does It Really Make a Difference? 14
Type O 16,   *Type A* 18
Type B 21,   *Type AB* 23

3 SUB-TYPES 26
Type Oa 28,   *Type Ob* 29,   *Type Ao* 30
Type Ab 30,   *Type Bo* 31,   *Type Ba* 32

———————— 4 ABOUT FOOD .... 33 ————————
How to Eat 33
Do's and Don'ts and Words of Advice 36
What Not to Eat 40

———————— 5 MENUS .... 45 ————————
Type O Menu 46,   Type A Menu 54
Type B Menu 60,   Type AB Menu 66
Type Oa Menu 69,   Type Ob Menu 73
Type Ao Menu 77,   Type Ab Menu 81
Type Bo Menu 84,   Type Ba Menu 88

———————— 6 HOW TO CREATE YOUR OWN DIET 93
Type O 93,   Type A 96,   Type B 100
Type Ab 104

———————— 7 VITAMINS AND MINERALS .... 108 ————————
Vitamin A 110,   Vitamin B 112,   Vitamin C 119
Vitamin D 121,   Vitamin E 121,   Vitamin K 122
Calcium 122,   Chlorine 123,   Chromium 123
Cobalt 124,   Copper 124,   Iodine 124
Iron 124,   Lysine 125,   Magnesium 125
Manganese 126,   Nickel 126,   Phosphorous 126
Potassium ... 127,   Selenium 127,   Sulphur 128
Sodium 128,   Silicon 129,   Tryptophan 129
Zinc 129

— 8 VITAMINS AND MINERALS FOR BLOOD TYPES .... 131 —
Type O.... 131,   Type A 132,   Type B 133
Type AB 133,   Type Oa 134,   Type Ob 134
Type Ao 135,   Type Ab 136,   Type Bo 136
Type Ba 137

———————— 9 CHILDREN AND HEALTH .... 138 ————————
Each Child is Different 139,   The Type O Child 140
The Type A Child 141,   The Type B Child 142
The Type AB Child 143,   Family Menus 143

_ 10 HOME THERAPIES FOR SPECIFIC CONDITIONS .... 145 _

Acne 146,   Alzheimer's Disease 147,   Anemia 147
Anorexia Nervosa 148,   Arthritis 148
Asthma 149,   Blood Pressure (High) 149
Blood Pressure (Low) 150,   Bronchitis 150
Cancer . 151,   Circulatory Problems 152
Colitis (Krohn's Disease) 153,   Constipation 153
Eczema/Psoriasis/Allergies 154,   Eye Conditions 154
Gall Bladder Problems 155,   Gout 156
Heart Conditions 156,   Hypoglycemia 157
Insomnia 159,   Liver Ailments 159
Low Back Pain 160,   Migraine 160,   Neuritis 160
Prostate Conditions 161
Sore Throats/Sinus Conditions 161,   Ulcers 162
Urinary Tract Ailments 162

11 CANDIDA OR YEAST 163

Getting Rid of Yeast 164

12 CHILDREN'S DISEASES 166

Fever 167,   Common Colds 167
Sore Throats 168,   Tonsillitis 169
Asthma 169,   Stomach Aches 170

APPENDIX A DIAGNOSTIC PROCEDURES 171

Iridology 171,   Pulse Diagnosis 174

APPENDIX B CLEANSING THERAPIES 177

Why are Therapies Necessary? 177,   Acupuncture 179
Colon Irrigation 180,   Color Therapy 182
Cranial Moulding 182,   Fever Therapy 182
Footbaths 183,   Immersion Bath 183
Inhalation Therapy 183,   Massage 184
Music Therapy 184,   Osteopathic Manipulation 185
Poultices 185,   Reflexology 185
Shiatsu 186,   Structural Alignment 186

Bibliography 187

Index 191

With special acknowledgment to
Dr. Joseph E. Pizzorno, Jr.
President of John Bastyr College
of Naturopathic Medicine;
Dr. L.J.B. Cardinal N.D., D.N.B., M.D.,
Chairman of the National Board
of Naturopathic Examiners;
Dr. Jules Haran, M.D.; and all
those other practitioners at
the various centers.

INTRODUCTION

Why is This Happening to Me?

Most of us consider ourselves to be healthy. We are busy and active, and we contribute to life. We are absorbed in our work, our play, and our relationships. We are excited about being alive. Then, one day, we have an ache, perhaps in our back. It is a shock. "Why is this happening to me?" we ask. The backache interferes with our plans. Suddenly we become aware that our bodies could break down, and we begin to confront the notions of aging and death.

By explaining away the backache as a part of the natural process of aging, we have, however, limited our expectations of health for the rest of our lives. A man may one day lean toward the mirror to shave and find that his body is stiff as he returns to normal posture. He accepts this as normal for someone his age. He may also notice that he can no longer spring out of a chair. Rather, he leans on the arms and pushes himself up. This, too, becomes normal. A woman may lean over to pick up a book lying on the floor. On standing up she feels dizzy. She does not view this as unusual. This same woman may find it difficult to wake up in the morning. Coffee soon becomes her only recourse before going to work.

These changes in our health come about so gradually that we truly believe our bodies have always been this way. We forget what vitality and alertness feel like. Or, if we can remember, we look upon boundless resources of energy as belonging only to children. We believe that age conditions our health. It is normal for a forty-year-old to find loud music intolerable. It is normal for a sixty-year-old to puff after climbing a flight of stairs. It is normal for an eighty-year-old to slip into confusion from time to time.

But are these things signs of health? Are they all we can expect of life? Let us start by looking at a newborn baby. Do you remember the first time you saw a new baby? There before you lay a charming little thing, dwarfed by the bassinette in which she had been placed. You saw her a month later and already she was much bigger. By three months of age the child was too big for the bassinet and had to be moved to a crib.

At the moment of birth, the immune system is more alive than it will ever be again. Cells do not just replace themselves, they triple and quadruple themselves. The baby grows no matter what. Before birth, each new cell created was perfect. It replicated perfectly its father/mother cell. The fetus received its nourishment from the placenta. Indeed, the fetus was a parasite. It lived off its host (the mother). If the mother did not consume food that gave the developing human what it required, the unborn child extracted nutrients from the mother's body.

After birth, however, the baby no longer chooses in the same way. Mother now feeds the child. The choices that the mother makes will determine the child's eating habits and thus her nourishment for the rest of her life. That nourishment will, in turn determine the quality of health that she will experience at age twenty, forty, sixty, and eighty.

Let us examine the smallest component in the human body, the cell, in order to understand how our nourishment affects it. Our bodies are made up of trillions upon trillions of cells — well beyond the number of people that live on the planet earth. There are a billion skin cells alone. It is nothing less than a miracle that each cell knows what it is and must do in the body. Never does a kidney cell make a mistake and form itself instead into a liver cell. Cells are organized perfectly. What keeps them organized is DNA, the architect of the body. DNA exists in every cell. RNA, also part of each cell, carries out the plans of its architect sister. RNA is analogous to the workers on a construction site who carry out the architect's plans. RNA is what monitors cell division or mitosis. Every day of life, millions of cells are destroyed and millions of new cells are created to replace them. RNA makes sure that each new cell is an exact replica of the cell it is replacing. Each cell is a perfect clone of the cell that preceded it. Thus, at the level of the cell, birth are death are going on each day of our lives.

To replicate themselves perfectly when they divide, our cells need nourishment. While we were still fetuses in the womb, they reproduced as perfect cells. However, in life we have the opportunity to choose what we eat. We can drink mineral water or we can drink beer when we are thirsty. We can eat roast chicken or fried sausages when we are hungry. We can enjoy fresh cantaloupe or French pastry when we want a snack. If we do not pay attention to what we eat, we may nourish ourselves in such a way that cells become weakened. Weakened cells then create other weakened cells in their place. Numbers of weakened cells can create weakened kidneys, weakened lungs, or weakened immune systems.

Just as improper nourishment creates weakened cells, proper nourishment can strengthen cells. Even genetic weaknesses can be strengthened. Our body's architect, DNA, holds within itself our strengths and weaknesses. Though it takes much longer to strengthen genetic deficiencies, it is possible for the architect to change her plans. No matter what our physical conditions are, it is possible to nourish them in such a way that we can enjoy strong bodies and a life full of vitality. It is never necessary to accept passively either arthritis or asthma. It is as possible to run a marathon at sixty as it is at twenty and to think as clearly at eighty as at thirty. The American painter Grandma Moses demonstrated to all of us that old age can include a firm brush stroke rather than trembling hands and a vivid imagination rather than a wandering mind. We were all endowed at birth with the treasures of health and vitality. We have only to discover the keys to opening these gifts.

What Can I Do about It?

There are only two methods to repair the damage that has occurred in our cells: proper food and proper exercise. The word *proper* is important here. Each of us was created differently, and each of us has different body needs. Some people need a vegetarian diet in order to thrive, while others must have meat. Some people need heavy exercise in order to function at their maximum, while others need to do only some light swimming. It is crucial that each of us discover for ourselves what patterns of nutrition and exercise will best serve us. That sounds simple enough, but it is really a formidable task.

At dinner, for example, children might be served roast beef, potatoes, green beans, and carrots. For dessert there is apple pie and ice cream. To drink, they have a choice of milk or coffee. Notice that they eat what their parents serve. It is acceptable not to eat the apple pie, but only if they are already full. One of the children may be an individual who should not eat meat. His body cannot tolerate it. His cells become burdened with mucous and fat. His stomach does not have appropriate quantities of acid to digest meat. His sister may be unable to tolerate mucous-forming foods. Ice cream and milk will clog her system. By eating what is served without discretion, she weakens her body.

A woman discovers a lunchtime exercise class and feels invigorated following it. Afternoons at work are no longer exhausting. She decides to take up running as well and before the evening meal runs four miles. She encourages her husband to do the same. He buys running shoes and a jogging suit and joins her each evening. However, while she comes home filled with energy, ready to make dinner, and then go out afterwards, he is so exhausted that he must take a long nap following their run together.

Just as we are individuals with individual talents and skills, so we also have individual bodies with individual needs. It is essential that we find out what these needs are and that we nurture them. This book will help you to do just that.

1

COMMITMENT
TO HEALTH

Results of a Healthy Menu

Are you feeling as well as you should? Are you functioning at your top mental ability? Are you experiencing life to its fullest? Are you as successful as you can be in your work? Are you enjoying your family and friends?

If your answer to even one of these questions is no, you have a problem. That problem was created by you and can be corrected by you.

About four years ago I examined a young man from New York who had low blood sugar. At the time he held a minor position in a large advertising firm. Having followed my menu and exercise recommendations for about a year and half, he returned to me for his third re-examination.

"When I first came to you I was a nobody in an advertising firm, "he said." Today I own my own company. I have just received the largest account that anyone in the business on the East Coast has landed in the last eight years — even among the largest firms!

"When I first came to you I was tired and depressed most of the time. I knew I had potential but I just couldn't seem to demonstrate it. I found myself blaming the people at work who wouldn't notice me, my parents who didn't believe in me, or even my friends who didn't have the right contacts.

"Your menu has made me feel better and better. I have stopped blaming everyone for my problems and have solved them all myself. I have so much energy and enthusiasm for my work and my life, I cannot believe it! Neither can any of my competitors believe my success. Nobody my age has landed an account like the one I just signed in a very long time!"

Now some may say that this man was just lucky. He, however, doesn't think so. He is absolutely certain that correct eating has nourished every single aspect of his life. Getting control of his eating habits allowed him to get control of his life. Again and again I encounter people like this young man. Though he gave me credit for his remarkable accomplishments, he is the one who did all the work. No one is a victim of circumstances. Life is always under our own control. It is the belief that circumstances control us that keeps is stuck in a certain position. People who are overweight say, "I just can't lose weight, I've tried everything." They get what they believe. People who hate their jobs say, "Well, I hate it, but at least I have a job." Such a belief ensures that they will always hate their jobs and never find another. Miracles are always possible if we are willing to take responsibility for our lives.

When Mrs. C. first came to me she had suffered headaches for twenty years. She had been diagnosed as having arthritis in her hands, back, and neck. Her gall bladder had been removed, she had had surgery to correct a hiatus hernia, and she was thirty pounds overweight. She was tense and depressed and had a blood pressure of 172/100. Thirteen weeks later this lady returned to be re-examined. Her blood pressure had fallen to 130/80 and she had lost thirty pounds. She had not had a headache since her menu had changed, and the aches and pains in her neck and back had reduced so much that she was now doing housework for the first time in many years. And she was much calmer. This lady had made a remarkable commitment to change her life. She was over sixty years old and of Italian extraction. In order to follow her menu she had to give up pasta and most of her other tasty dishes. This was very difficult for her. But look at the tremendous gains she made in the process.

Mrs. T. came to me in her early twenties. Her body was weakened. She was fatigued, hypoglycemic, had a urinary infection, and vaginal discharge. In the past she had had a serious case of venereal disease, and she had been told that, as a result, her fallopian tubes were fused. Two different gynecologists had recommended a hysterectomy. I could guarantee her nothing. I could only advise her to follow a specific diet and take herbs and vitamins. It was up to her to follow these suggestions. She did so faithfully. Two years later she delivered her first child.

We create illness and we can make the corrections necessary to relieve it. Mr. N, a New Yorker, was fifty-five years old when he first came to me. He had just suffered a severe myocardial infarction or heart attack. It was expected that he would have more. After a year of following a new menu and taking vitamin supplements as well as following an exercise program, his EKG and blood work were normal. When he asked his cardiologist how this could be so, the doctor replied, "Only God could do that." This man is still healthy today. He is living a full life, running a business, and enjoying being a grandfather.

It is difficult to believe that such results are possible for people and yet they happen in my practice time and time again. For over thirty years I have watched people's lives completely transform after they make changes in their menus. Not only does their health improve, so does their position in life. Those who enjoy their work are promoted. Others stop what they are doing and start new careers. What we feed ourselves touches every cell in the body. This includes the cells of the brain where intelligence and creativity lie.

Heal Me, Doctor.

Before I go on to discuss specific measures available to you to restore your health to full vitality, I want you to examine honestly your attitudes toward illness. Some of you are victimized by illness. You are likely to say something like: "Poor me!" or "Isn't it terrible?" or "Just when everything was going great for me, look what happened!" Others of you enjoy your illnesses. You don't really want to give them up. You might say to your spouse, "I'm sorry, I just can't do that today. I'm not feeling well. Perhaps you can do it for me." Rather than changing your diet, you might say, "I can't do that. That would be much too difficult. I have to cook dinner for the rest of the family and they would never eat that kind of food. Why should I?"

Look at your own experience and discover which of these attitudes you hold. An understanding of these attitudes is on essential prerequisite to a program of restoring health. Although like many other habits these attitudes are probably unconscious, they still affect the results you will achieve.

I see two basic personality types again and again in my practice. The first type I call the power wielder. This person uses illness to control those people closest to him: his spouse, his children, his parents, and even his peers. He manages upsets by creating bigger and better headaches. The severe headache controls the rest of the family. Nobody is allowed to upset the power wielder. Everyone must be quiet. They may even cancel plans to stay home and look after him. His wife will not discuss his financial irresponsibilities when he has a headache. Being sick, then, becomes a way of solving problems.

While this behaviour may be acceptable in the family and even in society, it cheats the individual out of experiencing life. It causes such people to miss out on the joys of clear communication with children. Beautiful days are lost, travel opportunities are missed, and friendships are given up. Certainly the person who behaves this way gets considerable amounts of attention, but the attention he receives engenders anger and resentment. He misses out on love and joy and excitement.

The second personality type is the individual who comes into the clinic and throws her money on the table. "I don't care what it costs. Heal me, doctor." This person takes no responsibility whatever for her health state. She treats her body like a machine. When it breaks down she goes to the mechanic and orders him to fix it up. It is as if her body were the family car. She knows perfectly well that one day the mechanic will not be able to fix the car, but then she will just buy a new one. What she forgets is that her body is the only one she will ever have. She cannot buy a new one. Putting all her faith in a doctor is like betting every cent she has at the race track. Never give up your participation in regaining health. In fact, money cannot buy your health, only your attention and commitment can do that.

An example of how subtly the mind works in these matters is all too familiar to those who run long distances. At some point in their run — it can be at the beginning, after three miles, after ten miles, or after twenty miles — the mind will begin to chatter away. "Oh, my knee is hurting, I really should stop," or "This is just too far to run today. I have much too much to do and not enough time for this," or "I hate running in the rain. Maybe I should stop and run twice as far tomorrow when it is sure to be a nice day." If the runner succumbs to these thoughts, he will stop his run and will not achieve the results he wants.

The obstacles to restoring your health are similar. You have developed many attitudes and habits and these keep you health at the same level. Each of these attitudes and habits can be rationalized. You may have resigned yourself to having arthritis because your mother, grandmother, and aunt all have arthritis. You believe that there is nothing you can do about it. You therefore accompany this illness with either resignation or anger, and these attitudes become part of your personality. People then respond to you according to that personality, and they, no doubt, reinforce your beliefs. They may say, "Isn't is terrible about Joan? What a lot of pain and suffering she has to bear," or they may say, "Gee, Joan is in a bad mood today. It makes it difficult for us to work with her. But then, she is suffering a lot of pain. We need to understand that." People will make excuses for you. They will expect less and less of you and ultimately you will do less and less until you are an invalid.

Our attitudes can trap us into keeping an illness. We must learn to recognize the thoughts that accompany them. A thought like, "Gosh, this diet is difficult. I must be crazy to be doing this," is attached to an old attitude or habit. There will always be good reasons that we don't want to change our diets. We have eaten in a particular way for ten, fifteen, twenty, forty, or even sixty years. This method has become ingrained in our bodies and is part of our belief system. Our taste buds have adjusted, and our friends and families expect it. What we need to remember is that the habit is what caused our illness. The one person who will always make the difference in the level of wellness you achieve is you. No doctor heals you.

Every day we live is a day of our life lost. As we grow older we realize that each day is precious. At one point you may ask: "Am I enjoying life?" If you are not, you probably have one of the following reasons:

1. *Because I am not healthy.*

2. *Because I cannot express myself in my work.*

3. *Because I don't have enough money.*

4. *Because I am not creative.*

5. *Because I don't have a relationship.*

6. *Because I don't make a difference in the world.*

All these problems can be cleared up when you take responsibility for your life. When you do that, when you realize that it is your life, not your mother's or your father's or your boss's or your child's, you have the opportunity to change your experience. It is you who expands your life. It is you who gets more money or more friends or better health. Change can be uncomfortable and it can be difficult, but if you are willing, you can have what you want. It is all up to you.

Is It Really All up to Me?

The thought that we might be responsible for the success or failure of our health restoration program is uncomfortable for most of us. We have grown up with the belief that germs or genes cause most illnesses and either there is a medicine to cure them or there isn't. These are convenient points of view, since they mean we do not have to take responsibility for our health. Whatever happens, either illness or health, it is caused by agents outside ourselves. In fact, in our mouths are enough germs to kill us. We do not develop illnesses because our immune systems are vital, active, and functioning well. When our immune system weakens, these same germs become active and create illness.

Naturopathic healing aims at the very source of an illness — at the weakened cells that created the overload on other cells. Because it has taken many years for the body to break down, many years of improper eating and improper exercise, healing is slow. Depending upon the severity of the condition, the age of the patient, and how much he is willing to do, the natural way of healing could take eight months or three years. However, repair is possible.

The essential ingredient in that repair is you. The doctor does not take your recommended supplements for you. He or she does not buy food for you, cook for you, or do your exercise for you. These things are entirely up to you. And these are the things that must be changed to restore your body to its full potential.

In the following chapters there is enough information for you to develop your own health program. Sticking to it is entirely up to you. But if you do so, you will be creating the best possible insurance policy for yourself. You will be creating an exciting and rewarding life for yourself, one filled with vitality, creativity, mental alertness, and boundless physical energy. One should not start any diet without the approval of his or her doctor.

Breaking Food Habits

You probably know that your eating and exercise habits need changing. Now you must ask yourself whether you are willing to do what it takes to shift gears into vibrant health.

You have established many comfortable habits over the years. Are you willing to give them up? Are you willing to transform your lifestyle? Most of you probably answer yes to those questions. My suspicion, however, is that you want someone else to do the work. This is not possible. Your body belongs to you, and your health is your most valuable treasure. Do not give up your responsibility for that health easily. No doctor can heal you. Only you can heal yourself. I cannot say this often enough.

Just a few days ago I was examining a seventy-nine-year-old man and seventy-two-year-old woman. He was a retired aircraft engineer from Montreal and now lived in a retirement hotel. She was a widower. As they were to be married in two weeks time, she decided they needed healthy diets. This elderly couple have clearly decided to create health and therefore a future for themselves.

Mrs. H. came to me following the removal of a lung. She was fatigued and stressed with a hacking cough. Even though it was clear that her smoking habit had caused her illness, she was unwilling to give it up. When I asked her why she would not give up smoking, she answered, "Because I am entitled to one comfort in my old age." This lady saw herself as old and yet she was only age fifty! She had no vision of herself as a vital, alive fifty-year-old.

No matter what your age, in order to be successful in changing your lifestyle you must have commitment. You must be committed to your menu and your exercise plan. You will be entering into a major readjustment in your life. Such an undertaking does not come easily. In order to find the foods suggested to you on your new menu, you may need to shop differently. It may be necessary to go to a health food store, a fish market, a fruit and vegetable market, and a butcher. At first it will seem as though you don't have enough time to do all of this. In fact, that may even be true. You will simply have to find a way to do these things anyway. There will be lots of good reasons for not following your menu. It may be expensive, inconvenient, time consuming, or awkward in social situations. All of these things are probably true. In order to be healthy, you will need to hold to your vision of yourself as healthy, and do them anyway. Recognize that when you listen to all your excuses for not giving up a habit, you are left with all the irritating conditions you say you don't want.

The difficulty in changing menus is that we are as addicted to food as drug addicts are to drugs. This addiction has developed almost from birth. Just as the drug addict needs a hit, many of us need our 3 P.M. snack, which, according to television commercials, consists of a chocolate bar or soda pop. If we don't have it, we develop the 3 o'clock blues.

Giving up a habit is consistent with loving yourself, seeing yourself as deserving the very best. Concentrating on your weaknesses will never help you to give up a habit. Rather than focusing on giving up junk foods, focus on eating proper foods. Again and again, when confronted with food, ask, "Now, which of these foods will support my body?" When you find that particular food, eat it. Concentrate on eating proper foods. Make your habit one that will allow you to get what you want out of life. You always own your habits. Be committed to owning good ones.

2

BLOOD TYPES

Blood Type — Does It Really Make a Difference?

If you have donated blood, had children, entered the armed services, or had surgery, your blood has been typed and you should know if you have O, A, B, or AB type blood. Most of us do little more with this knowledge than compare notes with friends and relatives to find out what type they are. We think nothing more about it. Yet our blood type is as integral to our individuality as our personality.

Although scientific studies of blood types and illnesses are only just beginning, there is already considerable evidence that certain diseases are more common among one blood group over another. For example, Type A's are found to have a higher incidence of gastric cancer than type O's. Type O's, on the other hand, have a higher incidence of both peptic and duodenal ulcers. While Type A's have a higher frequency of uterine cancer than other blood groups, Type O's have a higher incidence of toxemia.

There are, then, significant differences in the diseases that those in different blood groups develop. Little work has yet gone into researching why this may be. It may be that the answer lies in how the blood carries nutrients. Blood, after all, reaches every cell of our body. It transports nutrients and oxygen to all parts, keeping us alive. It also removes waste materials and takes them to appropriate locations for excretion. Carbon dioxide, for example, is taken to the lungs.

When I was studying to become a naturopath, my teachers believed that everyone should be a vegetarian. I traveled across North America and Europe, working with many different naturopaths and homeopaths. All of them insisted that we should all give up flesh foods. Not only did they believe that it was unnatural to kill animals, they concluded that human beings were not meant to be meat eaters. The natural carnivorous dog has a short bowel, while the human has a twenty-eight-foot intestine. All carnivorous animals have pointed, sharp teeth designed for tearing and chewing, while the human has teeth designed for mashing. And, finally, because blood contains waste products and meat contains blood, humans should not ingest flesh.

When I began my own practice, I assumed that my teachers were correct and advised all my patients to move toward a vegetarian diet. Nearly all patients did well initially. I suspect that these improvements related to the fact that most of them had also given up junk foods. However, after a period of time I had to face the fact that some patients did not do well on a vegetarian diet. I began to wonder whether some people were simply not suited to such a diet — a very uncomfortable thought since it contradicted all my education.

I had once worked as a blood technician with a pathologist who was investigating the relationship between the incidence of cancer and the structure of the red blood cell. His view was that if the red blood cell had a drum-stick look to it, there was a possible cancer in the body. That experience led me to the notion that perhaps blood was a critical factor to the health of an individual. I began to listen to my patients' concerns about their diets more carefully. I also began to notice that those with type A blood were thriving on the vegetarian diets. Those with type AB also did well. Individuals with Type B blood did less well and those with Type O found it impossible to remain on the diet. I noticed also how each type responded to exercise. Type O's were physical beings, while type A's were considerably less so.

Based on my observations I developed diets and exercise programs for each of the blood groups. Soon my patients began to respond to their new programs. The individual wants and needs of their bodies were being met directly, with remarkable results. Their vitality returned and clarity of mind was increasingly evident.

Let us look now at the four main blood groups — O, A, B, and AB. In the next chapter, we will look at the six subgroups that show up on the cusp of each main groups and combine the traits of two types. These I call Oa, Ao, Ob, Ba, Bo, and Ab.

Type O

Approximately 70 percent of the people in the world have Type O blood. These people have very physical bodies. The road to health for them is through physical exercise. Only through exercise can they truly release stress and tension. Talking helps them let go of tension, but physical exercise benefits them for more. A Type O individual, if he looks back into his childhood, will recall how physical exercise made him feel better. When he got upset with mother for not allowing him to go to a movie, he probably got on his bicycle and rode furiously down the road. He then quickly forgot his mother and joined some friends in a game of baseball. The desire to go to the movies had disappeared from his consciousness.

Type O's are revitalized by exercise. Their minds are stimulated by physical movement. If a Type O student is studying for an examination, she should first spend about an hour exercising. Before writing her examination, she is better off running or playing a game of squash than sitting down to study. Clarity of mind will come to her in this way and she will do better on the exam than she otherwise would have.

As problems arise, the Type O solves them best as he exercises. Problem-solving will be accelerated, and the individual will come to a faster resolution of the issue than if he pored over the information. Admittedly, such remarkable results for the Type O person only occur when he is in perfect health. Unfortunately few of us can claim to be in this condition. However, exercise is one of the crucial elements of a health-repair program for a Type O.

All matter is made up of atoms and molecules in perpetual motion. Thus, though it does not appear that way to us, our bodies are constantly in motion, constantly vibrating like an engine that idles. The Type O person has the highest idling speed of all blood types. Just as the engine idling on high burns more energy than one idling on low, so too does the Type O require high energy food. Being higher in protein, flesh foods fulfill this requirement. There is nothing higher in vibration than flesh.

Eating flesh goes against the beliefs of some religious groups and troubles many people concerned about chemical additives to meat. It is not my purpose to oppose religious beliefs. Concerns about chemicals are quite another matter. One must weigh the consequences of no meat to the Type O body versus the harm chemical additives may do to it. It is certainly possible to be wise about additives. Pork should be avoided. It is contaminated with both chemicals and bacteria. Beef is not advisable because it is injected with steroids and chemicals. Veal should also be avoided because calves are forced to eat chemical-laden food. Chicken, turkey, and fish (except tuna and swordfish, which contain mercury) are generally safe to eat.

Another danger faces the meat eater: she may not use up her food. Let us look at the diet of a normal office worker who leads a sedentary life. She gets up, has breakfast, spends a day at the office working very hard, comes home mentally exhausted, eats dinner, and then watches televison. Her breakfast consisted of toast, an egg, and coffee. At lunchtime she had a ham and cheese sandwich, a salad, coffee, and cake. For supper she eats lamb chops with all the trimmings. But she has done nothing physical to burn up this high energy food. Now, something good will turn into something bad. If animal protein is not dispersed through physical exercise, it will cause unease and will adversely affect the internal organs. The body will use it against itself. This is not surprising. A boiler that is given fuel and frequently stoked will explode if the valve is not opened to release the energy produced. What allows meat to support the Type O is the transformation of the energy it provides into motion.

Unfortunately, there is a paradox in the Type O's nature. He is basically lazy. It takes tremendous strength of will for him to go for a run or play a game of tennis. He doesn't want to exercise. He is rather like a Model T Ford that needs to be cranked in order to get it going, but once it has started, it doesn't want to stop. Type O's are very difficult to stop once they get started. If a Type O decides to win something, once he gets started, he will very likely do it. This is, of course, assuming that the Type O is in excellent physical health.

Type O's are capable of running up to fourteen miles every day. However, a forty-five-year-old who has never exercised and has not run in the last twenty years will not be able to and should not run fourteen miles. Before beginning an exercise program, anyone should have an assessment from a qualified physician. Then she can start slowly. She might walk a city block three times a day for four days. The next four days she can increase her pace. Next she might alternate walking with jogging. Finally, she may run that distance and gradually extend the distances covered. Contrary to what we imagine, a Type O who runs up to fourteen miles every day will not be exhausted by the run. She will be invigorated by it. Her mind will be clearer than she can remember it being, and her creativity will be at peak performance. Problem solving ability and energy resources will be awesome.

The key to the Type O is protein. But, if protein is eaten every single day, then exercise must also be done every single day. Three days a week of racquetball will not serve the Type O. The body will experience biochemical explosions. If alertness is the goal, exercise is the way.

The importance of exercise for the Type O cannot be emphasized enough. Time and time again I examine people who have immense talent. Frequently even they do not realize it. What they experience as full mental clarity and full energy is all they know. They have nothing else to compare themselves with but their own experience. The Type O *must* exercise. He will not realize his full potential until he does.

Type A

The Type A person was born with creativite and intellectual prowess. He is primarily a mental person and has a formidable mind and a natural clarity of thought. The Type A is the thinker.

People with Type A blood are at the opposite end of the spectrum from Type O's. Where the Type O requires high energy food, the Type A needs low energy food. This is, of course, understandable when one considers the difference between the amount of energy required to exercise the body versus that required to exercise the mind. Whereas the Type O requires vigorous physical exercise, the Type A requires light exercise only. Whereas the Type O could swim 100 lengths of the pool, the Type A should swim only ten lengths. Heavy exercise is likely to cloud the Type A's natural mental abilities. Where the Type O should exercise before making a decision, the Type A is wise to "sleep on it." The Type A should never make a decision under stress. Clarity of mind and creativity come to the Type O through exercise. The Type A is born with clarity of mind as well as with vast resources of creativity. These are natural attributes.

Type A's often suffer from chronic sinus conditions, have frequent colds, and succumb to allergies. They chill quickly, cannot tolerate abrupt temperature changes, and are exhausted following a sauna or a hot bath. They tend to be hyperactive people, always jumping with energy. Indeed, people often remark on their seeming endless energy resources. However, rather than healthy vitality, this energy is really nervous energy provided by the nervous system and the thyroid. When they are questioned, Type A's will often admit to feeling fatigued or exhausted. To most onlookers, however, they never appear this way.

If a Type A decides to paint her house, she goes immediately to the paint store, buys the paint, comes home and begins painting. At completion she feels exhausted. Because of their need to "get going," Type A's deplete their bodies. The Type A, like the Type O, experiences a paradox. The Type O hates to exercise and needs to do so in order to reach maximum potential. The Type A, on the other hand, is always ready to do things, but in doing them she exhausts herself. Interestingly, the Type A tends to like to release tension through physical exercise. It is essential for her to learn that physical exercise will deplete her mental clarity. There are other methods that will, however, support her.

What then does the Type A need to do to reach his maximum potential? There are three essential areas that must be attended to: diet, exercise, and environment.

The Type A body is a low-harmonic body, the polar opposite of the Type O. Thus, food for a Type A must also be low harmonic. Because the Type A has a much lower output of hydrochloric acid, he has a great deal of difficulty in digesting both dairy and meat products. Similarly, highly acidic foods create difficulty for the Type A. Whole-wheat products, which we typically think of as good for us, are composed of 80 percent acid. Apples are also highly acidic. These foods should be avoided.

Though a Type A's goal should be to become vegetarian, it is not wise to do this all at once. To begin with, one should avoid pork and beef. One might then move from hard cheese to soft, from whole milk to 2%. Breads such as sprouted wheat or soya should be eaten. Carrots must be well boiled before being included in a meal. Slowly the truth will take hold in the body. Though at first it may seem like the individual's lifestyle is becoming limited, the result to the body will be doors opening to creativity, health, and vitality.

Exercise for the Type A should be far less vigorous than that recommended for the Type O. Passive exercises, like Yoga and T'ai Chi, are excellent, and, for the elderly, slow walks. The primary strength of a Type A is in the mind. Too much exercise will cause a loss of sharpness. Athletes who are Type A's are usually thoughtful competitors. They are masters at strategy. Professional tennis players who are Type A's would probably play a game of technique and strategy while the O's would probably play a powerful base line game. The O athlete can count on his brawn to win. The A athlete will overcome his wiry body by using his brilliant mind to outsmart his opponent. I am reminded of a professional basketball star who had Type A blood. He told me that uses his mind to give him an edge on the court. He always knows where his teammates are, where opposition players are, what the likely odds are of this move achieving that effect, what angle the shot needs to be from this position.

The Type A need to stretch muscles and lengthen them. in elongating the muscles, she gets rid of stress in the skeletal muscular system. Heavy physical exercise shortens and tones muscles, but yoga and T'ai Chi stretch muscles.

Yoga and T'ai Chi also offer the kind of environment that supports the Type A. These exercises are a form of meditation, stilling the nervous system and all of the erratic energy that an A can exhibit. Type A is a delicate, finely tuned individual. If we were to describe a Type O as muslin, strong and adaptable, we would describe the Type A as fine french lace, delicate and intricate. In order for an A to release his creativity, he needs to surround himself with calm, tranquil people. He needs a quiet environment with soothing colors. He does not need the world to give him stimulation. Stimulation comes from within himself.

One towering intellectual of our time was George Bernard Shaw. He lived alone in the country and would often take long, slow walks. When he was in his mid-twenties he announced that he had become a vegetarian. The doctors of Harley Street told him that he would soon die on such a diet. George Bernard Shaw lived well into his nineties and was alert and productive until his death, which, by the way, occurred much later than the Harley Street doctors' deaths. It would be interesting to find out whether this immensely talented and formidible intellect was a Type A. He exhibits all the patterns for such an individual. He ate no meat. He lived in the tranquility of the country and his favourite exercise was walking. Notice, too, that his gifts were of the mind.

Such a lifestyle looks like an arduous one for a member of our meat-eating, chaotically busy, exercise-obsessed Western society. However, one can order fish when out at a restaurant. One can practice yoga. And one can make one's home one's private and tranquil castle if one so desires. The rewards to the Type A who does these things are monumental. Who can quibble with the accomplishments of a George Bernard Shaw?

Type B

Type B is the balance between the extremes of Type O and Type A. A much smaller group of the population then either O or A, these people are fascinating. The Type B has a stillness of both body and mind that neither Type O's nor Type A's possess. It gives him the ability both to listen carefully and to act decisively. Type B's make wonderful pyschologists since people love to tell them their problems. Sometimes I think that Type B's were created to be mediators between Type A's and Type O's. The fact that they are simultaneously mental and physical gives them the capacity to understand both extremes of the blood-type continuum without effort.

They are, at the same time, both creative and practical. I am reminded of a patient who began work as an engineer. Later he shifted careers and became a successful designer of ladies lingerie. Remarkably, he did not have a business manager. He knew innately how to run a business.

Type B's are orderly and organized. They keep their homes and work places tidy, and are an asset to any organization. In addition to intuitive managerial ability, they have the ability to weigh situations accurately. They like to know everything that is going on, and they have the ability to motivate people.

Several years ago, a well-to-do, successful businessman came to me for treatment. He brought his whole family to the clinic and all received excellent results from their programs. To reward his key personnel for the work they had done for him, he arranged for them, too, to be examined at my clinic. Remarkably, it turned out that all five of these people had Type B blood. With such support, his business could not have failed.

Type B's need to be at the center of an organization. A Type B who is a typist in an insurance company would never be fulfilled. She needs to be in a position to make decisions and develop stategies. If she were nourished in this way, she would in turn nourish the company.

Because she sits in the middle between the Type O and A, the Type B is initially somewhat more difficult to treat. She is of neither the vegetable kingdom nor the meat kingdom. She is a little of both. Often the determination arises out of past illnesses. If she has suffered from sinus problems, allergies, or circulatory difficulties, she should reduce her dairy intake. If she finds herself to be fatigued, she ought to increase the amount of protein she is taking. The healing process, then, will probably lean toward either the A vegetarian diet and passive exercise or the O diet, which includes flesh foods and active exercise.

As the B Type moves toward her full health potential, she will become like a well-oiled machine, a smooth interplay between the mental and the physical. She will benefit from both active and passive exercise, perhaps some yoga on rising, then, later in the day, a two- or three-mile run. Her diet will be both of the meat kingdom and the vegetable kingdom. Where the O Type gets little benefit from yoga and the A Type is unable to enjoy heavy physical exercise, the Type B is able to do both. The O Type thrives on meat and wastes away on a vegetarian diet. The A Type thrives on the vegetable kingdom and is burdened when eating meat. The Type B, however, is truly able to experience the best of both worlds!

Type AB

Type AB individuals lie somewhere on the continuum between Type A and Type B, but they often have strong leanings toward either Type A or Type B. If there is a leaning toward Type A, then the individual is more mental. A quiet and peaceful environment is required in order for that mental creativity to be released. Since the nervous system is the crucial one to these Type AB's, they should solve problems when they are most relaxed, never when under stress. If there is a leaning toward Type B, the individual finds himself attractive to people. People like being around him. As a result, he finds that people are always willing to do things for him. He is a valuable asset in an organization.

The Type AB individual possesses the innate creativity of the Type A along with the quality of order of the Type B. These qualities are of course, combined in various quantities. Two of my patients provide excellent examples. Both are highly creative, though each uses that creativity differently, probably because one leans more to the A and the other leans more to the B. The woman who leans towards the A Type is a poet. She has considerable mental and creative capacities. She is a productive writer because she and her husband live in an isolated part of the country where few people bother them. She makes sporadic visits to cities whenever she has a reading to give. Otherwise, she is a woman of the wilderness.

The other woman is a gregarious, outgoing person. She has many friends and acquaintances. She is an interior designer and is well known for her shrewd business deals. Obviously, she is the one who leans toward the B Type, for she has an excellent business sense and the ability to communicate well with others. Interestingly, too, she finds it necessary to do physical exercise every day. The poet, on the other hand, finds that walks in the forest surrounding her home are adequate for her. She practices yoga. Notice, however, that both women work in areas of considerable creativity. This is natural for them.

Leanings toward A or B are very individual. One person may be 20 percent A and 80 percent B, while for another the ratios may be 60 percent A and 40 percent B. Anyone who has Type AB blood should carefully read the sections concerning both Type A and Type B bloods in an effort to find his particular leaning. Some of the points raised in these sections should feel familiar to the Type AB.

Answering the following questions will also help the Type AB determine where he sits between A and B:

1. *Do you feel exhausted following physical exercise?*
2. *Do you feel sleepy following a hot bath or a sauna?*
3. *Are you upset by hyperactive people?*
4. *Do you have frequent sinus problems and colds?*
5. *Do you have circulatory problems?*

If your answers were yes, you probably have leanings toward the A blood type and should read the section on Type A blood. Dairy products should be dramatically reduced and probably eliminated altogether. Whole-wheat bread should be replaced by sprouted wheat. Fish and chicken can be tolerated.

If you answered no, you probably lean toward Type B and should read that section. Reduce the percentage of dairy products you comsume. Perhaps move to skim milk and soft cheeses. As well as fish and chicken, you may occasionally eat lamb and veal.

If you find yourself in the middle between A and B (you would have answered some of the questions with a yes and some with a no), you may have fish and fowl three or four days a week. Soft cheeses may be eaten two days a week. Whole wheat or rye bread may be eaten three days a week while sprouted wheat should be eaten on other days.

The kind of exercise that usually works for the Type AB is twenty minutes of yoga on rising to center the body and fifteen minutes of physical exercise after work each day to release tension.

3

SUB-TYPES

My research into blood types started in 1957. After I had treated thousands of patients according to their blood types, I felt I acquired enough knowledge and information to share it with the world. In 1980, I wrote *One Man's Food,* which gave me the opportunity to view my work with a fresh outlook.

One of my patients at the time was a famous photographer. He had been typed as Type O, yet he showed few of the normal Type O traits. In fact, he showed many of the characteristics of a Type A. He could tolerate neither heavy exercise nor dairy products. He was exceptionally creative, indeed had been internationally acknowledged as a master in his art. My book being fresh off the press, this situation was, of course, uncomfortable to me because he did not fit the picture I had just described. I decided to look at his blood, this time with the aid of a magnifying glass just to make sure that I had not made an error in the initial typing.

To type blood we use two sera, the yellow B serum and the blue A serum. When blood comes in contact with these sera, it either clots or it doesn't. If the blood does not clot when in contact with either blue or yellow sera, the individual is an O blood type. If the blood clots in the blue serum but not the yellow, then the individual is an A blood type. If the blood clots in the yellow serum but not the blue, the individual is a B blood type. If it clots in both, then the individual is an AB blood type.

When I tested my patient's blood again, I noticed that the blood in contact with the blue serum was clotting finely all around the perimeter. Since most of the blood remained unclotted and the blood in contact with the yellow serum was unclotted entirely, he was certainly an O blood type. However, that clotting perimeter suggested that his blood did, in fact, contain traits of what I call A-type blood. Thus I discovered that though an individual might be one blood type overall, he might also have tendencies toward an entirely different blood type. That would explain this man's tendencies toward the A-type.

Clearly my patient required an entirely different diet than that of the straight Type O. Since he had highly dominant A characteristics, I treated him as what I came to call a Type Oa.

As I developed this concept over the next five years in my work with more than 3,000 patients, I was finally able to explain abberations that had appeared in my former patients: Type A's who loved sports, Type O's who could not tolerate noisy, busy environments, and Type B's who preferred to be alone. Gradually, six sub-types were identified: Type Oa, Type Ob, Type Ao, Type Ab, Type Bo, and Type Ba. Incredibly, my patients, too, felt comfortable with the notion, and the success rates of their programs jumped forward remarkably. It was as if I had finally found the missing pieces in a jigsaw puzzle.

Sub-types probably appear because an individual's parents have different blood types. For example, a father with Type O blood and a mother with Type B blood might produce an Ob child. But there is nothing clear about a sub-type. It is a matter of percentages. Some individuals may be 80 percent Type O and 20 percent Type A, while others will have a 60/40 ratio. Moreover, it is very difficult to identify leanings without carefully examining a person's blood. My hope is that the following information will allow you to adjust your program so that it will become more your own.

Type Oa

The photographer I just mentioned who had Type Oa blood clearly had a high ratio of Type A. He was first and foremost creative, he was exhausted following physical exercise, and he could not tolerate dairy products.

If you are a Type O, you can identify yourself as an Oa by answering yes or no to the following questions:

1. *Were you subject to colds as a child?*
2. *Do you or have you suffered from allergies?*
3. *Do you suffer or have you suffered from sinusitis or asthma?*
4. *Do you have thyroid problems?*
5. *Does reading entice you more than physical exercise?*
6. *Do your extremities become cold frequently?*
7. *Do you feel fatigued after exercise?*
8. *Do you have any allergies to dairy products?*
9. *Have you had problems with your gall bladder?*
10. *Are you creative?*
11. *Do you suffer from arthritis?*
12. *If you are a woman, do you have a vaginal discharge?*
13. *Does a sauna or hot bath fatigue you?*

If you answered yes to six or more of these questions and have been told you have Type O blood, you are probably an Oa Type. Thus, it is probably unwise for you to be involved in a fourteen-mile run. Four to six miles may be okay. However, you would be wise to introduce small amounts of yoga into your daily routine. Dairy consumption should be avoided at first, then slowly reintroduced into your diet. If you develop a mucous condition, then reduce dairy poducts again, ultimately reaching about half the amount of a normal O. Only veal, chicken, and lamb should be eaten with a heavy emphasis on fish. It is essential too, that you read the section about Type A. Between 20 and 50 percent of the Type A segment regarding the mind is applicable to you.

Type Ob

This individual possesses most of the qualities of an O Type as well as 20 to 50 percent of the qualities of a B. He probably has considerable clarity of mind as well as a great deal of creativity. I can think of two people who bear this blood type. One is a woman who spent twenty years as a nurse, ultimately becoming a director of a hospital. Then, one day she quit. She now writes, teaches English to first-year college students, and studies classical guitar. The other is a man who spent twenty years as a monk. He, too, left that work and now spends time with people as a counselor and simultaneously pursues a career as a pianist. Each person has diverse talents and abilities. But notice too that they are involved with people, the one as a teacher and the other as a counselor. They both have strong B leanings. If you have been told you have Type O blood, answering the following questions will indicate whether you are a Type Ob.

1. *Are people easily attracted to you?*

2. *Do people often try to tell you their troubles?*

3. *Do you enjoy working in the center of an organization?*

4. *Do you suffer from some type of allergy?*

5. *Do dairy products disagree with you?*

6. *Could you tolerate being a vegetarian?*

7. *Would you rather read a book than run?*

8. *Do you have a broad range of seemingly unrelated interests?*

9. *Does disorder upset you?*

If you answered yes to four or more of the questions or more than those for the Oa, you are probably a Type Ob and should read the section on Type B. You should reduce your dairy intake, but you can handle flesh foods. Fish, chicken, veal, lamb, and occasionally beef can be eaten. Physical exercise is essential for you.

Type Ao

The Ao Type fits somewhere along the same continuum as the Oa. Interestingly, there are fewer Ao's than Ab's. The Ao's are normally very physical people. I am reminded of a successful businessman who stays in the city during the week, but who feels that it is essential for him to leave it on weekends. In winter he skis and in summer he sails. He also enjoys competition and plays tennis in summer, squash in winter. His desire to win has been a great asset to him in business. If you have been told you have Type A blood, the following are questions that will help you to identify yourself as an Ao:

1. *After three months of a vegetarian diet, do you experience fatigue?*
2. *Does heavy physical exercise invigorate you?*
3. *Are you bothered by colds or sinusitis?*
4. *Do you feel fatigue following a sauna or hot bath?*
5. *Does physical exercise stimulate your mind?*

If you answered yes to questions 1 and 2 and 5 and no to questions 3 and 4, you are probably an Ao Type. Read the section on Type O in order to understand yourself a little better. You will always need fish, chicken, lamb, and some veal. If your lifestyle is a highly physical one, you may need to eat flesh food every day. About fifteen to twenty minutes of yoga as well as ten to fifteen minutes of heavy exercise very day will be adequate for you.

Type Ab

This person has the Type A kind of energy but can function very well in making decisions. If you have been told that you have Type

A blood, here are questions that may help you identify yourself as a Type Ab.

1. *Do dairy products affect your body?*

2. *Did you have frequent colds as a child?*

3. *Do you enjoy running a business?*

4. *Do you enjoy group situations?*

5. *Are people attracted to you?*

6. *Are you able to communicate ideas well?*

7. *Is there a need for you to do physical things?*

8. *Do you like order in your life?*

9. *Do you find it easy to get people to do things for you?*

If you answered yes to more than six of the above questions, you are probably an Ab, and you should read the section on Type B's. You may eat a small percentage of dairy products and can tolerate fish and chicken (mostly fish). Three or four days a week should be vegetarian. Though you do require physical exercise, you need less than that for the Type Ao.

Type Bo

This individual is highly physical. He can run ten miles per day and enjoys competitive sports. He is very enthusiastic, communicates well with people, and enjoys groups and organizations. He is the kind of person who can communicate better while exercising. If he were to carry out complex business negotiations, he would be best to do so on the golf course. He should always have access to a gym and should do physical exercise before making important decisions. If you have been told that you have Type B blood, questions that may help identify you as a Bo are as follows:

1. *Are you competitive in sports?*

2. *Do you enjoy discussing business while playing sports?*

3. *Do you have a strong leaning toward flesh foods?*

4. *Do you enjoy debates?*

5. *Do you solve problems while exercising?*

6. *Would you rather have a holiday that included vigorous sporting activities than one which consisted of lying on the beach?*

If you answered yes to four or more of these questions, you are probably a Type Bo. Dairy products can be enjoyed with minimum cutbacks and flesh foods can be tolerated very well.

Type Ba

These people possess all the qualities of the B-type and, added to those, have considerable reservoirs of the Type A creativity. In childhood these people may have had many colds. They may, in adulthood, suffer from circulatory problems and allergies. If you have been told that you have Type B blood, answering the following questions will help you identify yourself as a Type Ba.

1. *Do you reach decisions when most relaxed?*

2. *Do quiet environments help you make decisions?*

3. *Do hyperactive people upset you?*

4. *Do you prefer yoga to running?*

5. *Do you gravitate toward being a vegetarian?*

6. *Do you prefer subdued colors around you (blues and greens)?*

If you answered yes to four or more of the above questions, you are probably a Type Ba. Removing dairy products from the diet is essential to your well-being. Whole-wheat products need to be replaced by sprouted wheat and soya-based foods. Chicken, fish, and lamb can be tolerated. Exercise should be predominently passive in nature.

4

ABOUT FOOD

How to Eat

There are two essential ingredients to the menus I recommend. The first aspect is the content: that is, *what* foods should be eaten. These will be discussed in detail later. The second aspect is *how* these foods should be eaten: that is, what combinations of food allow for optimum digestion and thus provide optimum energy levels. This is perhaps the most difficult part of my menus for most people. We all realize that fresh fruits and vegetables, unprocessed meat, and unsalted nuts are good for us. What we rarely consider is how food is digested and the implications of that on eating.

Once food enters the body it is chemistry. Sugar's chemical name is CH_2OH. Protein is composed of carbon, hydrogen, oxygen, and nitrogen. It may also contain sulfur, phosphorus, iron, and cobalt. What you may think of as carrot, I think of as carotine. What you may think of as celery, I think of as sodium, since sodium is one of its major components. What you may think of as watermelon, I think of as silicone, one of its components. Understanding the chemical structures of foods helps determine how and what foods should be eaten. In order for digestion to take place correctly, exactly the right chemicals must be added to the food. Starch cannot be digested unless the right enzyme appears in the right medium.

Food provides us with energy. If the food is not digested properly, the body is deprived of its most vital element. If we do not chew our bread well, we fail to activate the salivary glands enough for appropriate quantities of ptyalin to be produced. Ptyalin, the enzyme that digests starches, is found in saliva. Starches that are well chewed move into the stomach with enough ptyalin to digest them in about two hours. Improperly chewed starches may remain in the stomach for up to five hours and even then may not be completely digested.

Ptyalin can only work in an alkaline medium. Even mild acids will inhibit its functioning. Thus one should never eat an acidic food alongside a starchy one. This seems easy enough. For example, apple pie is a combination of starch and acid. This favourite dessert, then, is difficult for digestion. Fruits and starches are not the only poor combination. Protein and starch are also hard to digest. The enzyme that initiates protein digestion — pepsin — is produced in the stomach and requires an acid medium in order to work. The ptyalin that initiates the digestion of starches requires an alkaline medium. When both enzymes — pepsin and ptyalin — are secreted together, they are both neutralized by the other's medium. The ptyalin encounters acid and the pepsin encounters alkaline. One of our favourite lunches, the meat sandwich, is thus not digested properly since it is composed of protein and starch.

The accompanying diagram gives you an excellent idea of proper food combinations. Vegetables, tofu, nuts, and seeds can be eaten with either animal proteins or with starches. However, animal protein should never be eaten with starch. Interestingly, that eliminates the mainstay of the North American diet: meat and potatoes. (I classify potatoes as a starch.) As fruits are acid or alkaline in nature, it is wise to eat fruits alone.

Changing our diet combinations is theoretically easy enough. It can, however, be difficult in practice. Because we have been combining our foods so that they slow down digestion, foods generally stay in the stomach for much longer than necessary. This extended period of food in our stomach has come to be interpreted by us as "feeling full" following a meal. When proteins are no longer combined with starches, the sensation of feeling replete changes. No longer do we experience a kind of heaviness. Because digestion is not inhibited, wastes are eliminated faster. Since foods are being

Food-Combination Chart

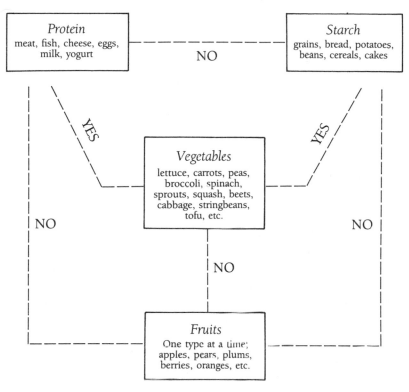

digested with greater ease, they leave the stomach sooner and so the stomach feels empty. At first we experience this change as meaning that we have not had enough to eat and we want a piece of bread or a sweet dessert. This addition to the meal slows down the digestive process, and we will feel that we have finished our meal. Only discipline and knowledge can break an individual of this habit. Eventually he does experience "feeling full" again. It is, however, a different feeling. It is a lighter and more complete feeling.

When we don't eat properly, we need large amounts of food to get enough nutrients. Furthermore, wrong combinations of foods will remain in the stomach longer than proper combinations. Improper eating, then, expands the size of the stomach. The stomach should be about the size of a clenched fist. Most people, because of poor eating habits, have expanded the size of the stomach. Such enlargement is certainly the cause of a such common complaints as hiatus hernias, perforated ulcers, gastric ulcers, or other stomach distress. Until the stomach shrinks to its healthy size, proper eating can leave one feeling hungry. Eventually, however, small quantities of food will be enough.

Though I cannot say for sure, I think this is one of the reasons many of my patients lose weight on the menus I recommend. They no longer use carbohydrates as a filler. For example, before treatment a patient's daily menu may consist of cereal, toast, and coffee for breakfast, a sandwich and fruit for lunch, and meat, potatoes, and a sweet dessert for supper. After starting a proper diet, the individual may eat a breakfast consisting of water and lemon juice, a half grapefruit, oatmeal, and herb tea. Lunch will be a salad of romaine lettuce, sprouts, cucumbers, celery, parsley, tofu, sesame seeds with a dressing of oil, lemon, and garlic. In addition, a piece of toast and an herbal tea will be taken. Supper will be made up of meat or fish with several vegetables. As you can see, the new diet has two fewer pieces of bread, and the potato and a sweet dessert are gone from the menu. Where snack time may have consisted of doughnuts and coffee, now snacks consist of a handful of almonds or a piece of fruit. When one combines foods so that they support digestion, large quantities of carbohydrates drop away.

I cannot emphasize enough the importance of combining foods properly. Eating in this way allows for digestion of food with ease. No longer will the body have to fight against itself to be properly nourished. This reduced strain on body processes will in turn make the individual more relaxed.

Do's and Don'ts and Words of Advice

Before making major changes to your diet, please remember that these require considerable changes in lifestyle. Most of us have been eating poorly all of our lives and are addicted to many foods. It is best to make changes carefully and slowly. For many people, rigidly adhering to a new menu overnight is very stressful. This stress is not needed by an already nutritionally stressed body. If it takes one to three months to ease into a new menu, no harm will be done. In fact, by adding a new dietary habit every week one can almost slip into a proper diet naturally!

Shopping

1. *Buy vegetables that are organically cultivated. If they are not available, use fresh or frozen, never canned vegetables. Organic foods are expensive but they are a wise investment for your future well-being.*

2. *Buy only vegetables indicated on your menu. Those not indicated should be strictly avoided.*

3. *Fish should always be fresh. When eyes are colourless and grey, the fish is not fresh or it has been frozen. There should be a bright red hue behind the gills. Never buy fish that has been filleted or that has had the head removed.*

4. *Tofu should be purchased from a health store. Cover it with water and store in the refrigerator. Change the water every day to keep it fresh. Use it before it becomes slippery, changes color or tastes sour.*

5. *Much of the meat available is tenderized with steroids. Whenever possible, buy free-range meat that has not been injected.*

6. *Organ meats are far better for the body than musculature because they are free of uric acid, which is common in muscle.*

7. *The harder the cheese, the higher the bacteria count. Thus, it is wise to eat softer cheeses.*

8. *Imported cheeses should be avoided because they contain more chemicals than most domestic cheeses.*

9. *Avoid tuna and swordfish as they contain large quantities of mercury.*

10. *Avoid lobsters, shrimp, and mussels because they are scavengers.*

11. *Salmon is best eaten in the summer. Winter salmon is usually fatty.*

12. *Codfish can be eaten in winter. In summer it swims closer to shore and contains a worm.*

13. *Buy only those fruit juices that are stored in glass containers and contain no added sugar or preservatives.*

14. *Read all labels when buying packaged foods. Avoid those containing preservatives either in the food or in the packaging.*

15. *Buy only fresh nuts. Nuts become rancid quickly.*

16. *Avoid iceberg lettuce. It contains minimal food value.*

17. *Buy only ungassed bananas. Bananas brought to North America from the Caribbean islands are picked unripened and are sprayed with natural gas for ripening when they arrive here. The chemistry of the banana is thus altered dramatically.*

Cooking

18. *Cooking utensils should be made from cast iron, porcelain, enamel, or corning ware. Avoid teflon, aluminum, and plastic utensils.*

19. *All vegetables should be washed thoroughly prior to cooking. Hold vegetables to the light to check for possible insects.*

20. *Never boil vegetables; they lose their nutritional value when boiled. Vegetables should be eaten raw or steamed. Purchase a steamer insert or a pressure cooker. For Type A blood, carrots must be boiled, but the water must be discarded as the carotine is much too concentrated.*

21. *When cooking for extremely ill patients, steam vegetables; these are more easily digested and passed.*

22. *Juice extracting machines should be used only after consultation with your doctor. Vegetables juices are highly concentrated and may have harmful effects.*

23. *Brown rice should be cooked with two teaspoons of nutritional yeast.*

24. *Dry soya beans should be soaked for twenty-four hours before cooking. During cooking the water should be changed each time a white film appears on it. This will prevent flatulence.*

25. *Never heat or cook natural honey because heating destroys the enzymes.*

26. *All oils should be fresh and stored in the refrigerator.*

Eating

27. *Never eat when nervous or tense. Even beneficial foods can work adversely under conditions of stress.*

28. *Never drink liquids that are too hot or too cold. Extreme heat and cold shock the body cells and interfere with the activity of the gastric juices.*

29. *Eat at least five green vegetables per meal. One quarter package of each frozen vegetable is enough for one meal.*

30. *Vegetables for breakfast? Yes, if you want.*

31. *Do not eat fruits directly before or after meals. Fruit should be eaten twenty minutes before or forty-five minutes after a meal.*

32. *Always wait thirty minutes after drinking vegetable or fruit juices before eating solid food.*

33. *Do not drink during a meal. Water and juices dilute digestive juices.*

34. *Nuts should be chewed thoroughly and should not be eaten in quantity. Peanuts and cashews are legumes (which are carbohydrates), not nuts (which are proteins).*

35. *Daily rations of vitamins and supplements should be spaced and taken with meals. Do not take more than recommended as too many may be detrimental. Use as little water as possible when taking vitamins and never take juices with vitamins. Take only prescribed vitamins. Vitamins are concentrated food substances, not drugs. Food may not be concentrated enough to revitalize the body so vitamins are prescribed only for periods necessary to do so.*

36. *Dried fruits can be eaten by all blood types if bought from a health food store and if the individual has no problem with sugar.*

Rules

37. *Do not mix a carbohydrate with a protein food during the same meal. Follow the food combining guide.*

38. *All lunches should be vegetarian.*

39. *Do not mix acid and alkaline fruits at the same meal.*

40. *Drink six to eight glasses of water every day. Drink tap water filtered through water purifiers attached to sink taps. Also recommended are glass-bottled mineral water and spring water, never carbonated or charged water. Water cleanses the kidneys and kidneys filter the blood. Water will help the kidneys to function at peak performance and prevent them from becoming diseased.*

41. *Do not eat sugar with a protein; for example, meat followed by a sweet dessert.*

42. *Fasting should be undertaken only after consulting your doctor. Fasting could be very shocking to the system if it is not fully cleansed. When no food is eaten, the body scavenges food from the colon. This creates fermentation in the system.*

43. *Exercise before eating, not after. We should rest after eating allowing the blood to circulate to the stomach for proper digestion. Exercise moves blood to the extremities and so will inhibit digestion.*

What Not to Eat

The quality of the food we eat affects the quality of our health. We are beginning to see that the old adage "you are what you eat" may not be so far off the mark. Research has now proven that high-cholesterol foods taken in excess contribute to heart conditions. Sugar has been demonstrated to be harmful to us. Even cow's milk has come into question. A calf fed pasteurized milk will soon die. The pasteurization process destroys vitamins and alters the original chemical structure of the milk. We know that white bread is, for the most part, depleted of all its vitamins. Even though it is attractive, it is non-nutritious. Preservatives being used in food as well as pest control sprays and chemical fertilizers are known to endanger health. All in all, the question of what we should eat is a confusing one to most people, even those who are following their idea of a natural diet.

Two foods we know that everyone should avoid, however, are sugar and coffee, two North American favourites.

Sugar

Sugar is a simple carbohydrate. Other such carbohydrates include brown sugar, honey, molasses, corn syrup, maple syrup, and synthetic syrups. On food labels they appear as sucrose, dextrose, or maltose. When these simple sugars are eaten, the pancreas quickly releases insulin to metabolize it. However, insulin remains in the bloodstream longer than the sugar, and the circulating insulin maintains blood sugar at a low level, even after the sugar that caused the insulin release has disappeared. This situation, if repeated often enough, will cause hypoglycemia, a condition presently plaguing North American society. Twenty to twenty-five years ago, people with this condition were sent to a psychiatrist, or they were encouraged to take extra sugar. Today much more is known about the effects of hypoglycemia. Conditions such as hyperactivity, inability to concentrate, loss of memory, and irritability are often caused by this problem. Hypoglycemia is the number one disease of this generation primarily because of our inordinate consumption of refined and processed foods.

Mrs. J. was fifty-eight years old when she came to me, complaining of exhaustion, depression, and an inability to enjoy her husband and children. In the morning she was tired, moody, and out of sorts until after she had had three or four cups of coffee. She and her husband were farmers, but as the years went on she could do less and less work on their farm. She had bouts of extreme exhaustion and constantly argued and fought with her husband and children. At one point she suffered from alcoholism and had undergone psychoanalysis. On examination she was found to be hypoglycemic.

Once Mrs. J. ate what was appropriate for her, her life changed dramatically. She was suddenly capable of doing more work on the farm than she had ever done in her life. But more important, her relationships with her husband and children transformed. Instead of fighting with them she laughed with them. She is astonished now when she looks back at her life to see what she missed. When the physical body works well, relationships work well.

But hypoglycemia is not the only problem arising from increased sugar consumption. The large amounts of circulating insulin in the bloodstream following the metabolizing of sugar may cause cardiovascular complications like atherosclerosis. As Durk Pearson and Sandy Shaw wrote in *Life Extension:*

Insulin suppresses growth hormone release and may, therefore, impair the immune system's ability to destroy atherosclerotic plaques, bacteria, viruses, and cancer cells. Since an important amount of growth hormone is released during the first hour and a half of sleep, it is particularly important not to eat table sugars or foods containing large quantities of it within a few hours of bedtime.

Sugar is a recent addition to our diet. Sugar factories did not exist until the nineteenth century. In 1850, total world sugar production was 1.5 million tons a year. In 1977, it was 70 million tons a year and growing. It has been demonstrated again and again that diabetes and heart disease increase at the same rate that sugar consumption increases. Dr. George Campbell has found that several diseases emerge when any culture increases its sugar intake dramatically: "diabetes, obesity, coronary thrombosis, gallstones, peptic ulcer, diverticulosis, varicose veins, hemorrhoids, E. coli infections, dental caries and, in part, cancer of the colon, hypertension, hiatal hernia and gout."

Sugar is the staple ingredient in processed food. If you examine labels on foods you buy, you will be astounded at the amounts of sugar you are eating. Canned tomato soup and canned beef consommé contain sugar. Peanut butter, packaged dry toast, and canned peaches contain sugar. So do dry breakfast cereals, ketchup, and tonic water. Not only do they contain sugar, however. Most of the long chemical names belong to preservatives. Aside from the fact that these additives may be hazardous to your health, they certainly complicate the process of digestion.

Coffee

Life sugar, coffee did not become a popular staple in diets until recently — the late eighteenth and early nineteenth centuries. Drinking coffee often goes hand in hand with sugar addition. Those who eat sugar at bedtime risk feeling exhausted when they wake up in the morning. The fatigue is created by the excess insulin in the bloodstream, and for most people today, it is counteracted by a cup coffee. Caffeine is a stimulant to the nervous system and gives the drinker artificially induced energy. If an individual alternates eating sweets with drinking coffee, he may seen to have constant energy. The coffee counteracts the fatigue caused by the insulin circulating in the blood after the sugar has been metabolized. Having a cup of coffee stimulates the nervous system so that energy will return. Notice, however, that the kind of energy that returns is nervous energy. This is no solution to low blood sugar.

Coffee is a poison. The caffeine in it is a dangerous narcotic drug belonging to the same alkaloid group of chemicals as morphine, nicotine, cocaine, and strychnine. Heavy coffee drinking can result in addiction. It frequently causes a serious Vitamin B_1 deficiency. Moreover, like any drug, in large doses it can cause an individual to become toxic. A healthy young person will excrete the nitrosomes and chlorogenic acids through her kidneys. However, with advancing age and less resiliant kidney functioning, these poisons will be retained by the body. Nitrosomes are possible carcinogens, and chlorogenic acids will inhibit cellular absorption of nutrients.

Along with these natural components in coffee, we receive the effects of deadly pesticides used by growers. For some twenty years now, Aldrin, Dieldrin, Chlordane, and Heptachlor have been used by Colombian coffee planters on their plants.

Nor is decaffeinated coffee safe to drink. Trichloroethylene, a close relative of the plastic chemical vinyl chloride, is used to extract the caffeine from coffee. Trichloroethylene is used mainly as a degreasing agent in the metal industry and as a solvent and dry-cleaning agent in the clothing industry. If it is used in this way in industry, what, then, could it do to our bodies?

Additives and Chemicals

Chemical preservatives, coloring agents, and artificial flavorings are common constituents of the foods we eat. Some of them, such as the nitrites added to meats to prevent discoloration, have been demonstrated to be virulent carcinogens.

The extent to which North Americans have increased their consumption of junk food is awesome. Between the years of 1959 and 1970 milk consumption reduced by 20 percent while soft drink consumption increased by 79 percent. When fruit and vegetable intake dropped by 50 percent, bakery product intake increased by 67 percent, potato chips by 85 percent, ice cream by 29 percent, and artificially flavored fruit punch by an unbelievable 750 percent.

Food, when it enters the body, is nothing more than simple chemistry. The body has been designed to manage the simple chemical structures that the earth provides. When these structures are compounded by complex chemicals, the body must work much harder to digest them. Improper digestion will always bring health problems.

Moreover, the longer food is stored, the greater the nutritional loss. Vitamins and minerals are often unstable and can be destroyed by freezing or overheating. In choosing to decrease our consumption of fresh fruits and vegetables and increase our consumption of processed foods, we are necessarily reducing the nutritional value of the food we eat. This will, in turn, alter our health state.

5

MENUS

Since I have been working with blood types, I have come across very few people who had a real intuitive sense of the foods that they required. Most of my patients, who had eaten to satisfy their taste buds, have accumulated high levels of toxicity and weakened their bodies. Since I could never recommend a diet based on a balanced state of health for these patients, I adapt a diet from the ideal state according to each patient's current physical condition.

Healing through nutrition is dynamic and ever-changing. A diet that I designed for you today in your current state of less-than-perfect well-being may no longer be right for you when, in the future, your body heals and achieves a state of balance. Diets have to be augmented, adding more foods to meet new physical needs, or reduced when certain foods are no longer required for their nutrient value.

Following are my recommended diets for each blood type in a perfectly balanced state of health. These diets are the ideal — the reality must be adjusted to each individual. Later I am going to show you how you can, by evaluating your current state of well-being and vitality, create a diet that will help you to achieve the state of health and energy you long for.

 *Type O Menu*

The Type O diet includes animal protein, the amount varying according to the amount of exercise the individual gets.

Meats

beef	duck	lungs
brain	heart	pheasant
buffalo	intestines	turkey
calf's liver	kidney	veal
chicken	lamb	venison

Fish

bass	herring	scrod
bluefish	mai mai	sea bass
brook trout	orange roughy	sea trout
cod	pickerel	skate
flounder	pike	sole
grouper	red snapper	turbot
haddock	salmon	white snapper
halibut		whiting

Eggs

four to five per week, boiled or poached

Cheese

Brie	farmer's	Munster
Camembert	goat	neufachtel
cheddar	gouda	provolone
colby	Gruyère	quark low-fat
cottage	havarti	ricotta
Edam	mozzarella	Swiss

__ Milk and Milk Products __

butter milk	skim	2%
goat's milk	soybean milk	yogurt
institute spread*	tiger's milk (available	rice milk
raw cow's milk	in a health food store)	

Recipe for Institute Spread: 1/4 lb. sweet butter }
1/4 c. safflower oil } *blend and*
1 Vitamin E capsule } *refrigerate*
1 lethicin capsule }

_____ Whole Grains _____

barley	kamut	pasta
brown rice	kasha	pilaf
buckwheat	millet	spelt
		wheat grains

_____ Vegetables _____

agar	dandelion greens	okra
alfalfa	daikon	olives
artichokes	eggplant	onions
asparagus	endive	savoy cabbage
avocado	escarole	seaweed (once a month)
bamboo sprouts	fennel	snow-pea pods
beans (all types)	fresh peas	spinach
bean sprouts	green rhubarb	squash (all types)
beets	kale	Swiss chard
beet greens	kelp	tomatoes
broccoli	kohlrabi	water chestnuts
carrots	leeks	watercress
celery	lentils	white cabbage
chick peas	lettuce (all types)	white corn
chicory	mushrooms	yeast
cucumber	mustard greens	yellow corn

Fruits

apples	dates	peaches
apricots	elderberries	pears
bananas (once a month)	figs	persimmons
blackberries	grapefruit	plums (dark Italian)
black grapes	guava	pomegranate
blueberries	honeydew melons	raisins
bread fruit	kiwi	raspberries
cantaloupe	lemons	star apple
cherries	limes	strawberries
coconut	mangoes	tangerine
currants (occasionally)	oranges	watermelon
custard fruit	papaya	

Fruit Juices

apple	cherry	orange
apricot	cranberry	papaya
blueberry	grape	water and lemon
carrot (occasionally)	grapefruit	

Cereals

bran	Grapenuts	rice bran
cornmeal	millet	shredded wheat
cream of whole wheat	oat bran	soy flakes
Familia	oatmeal	soy granules
5-grain	puffed rice	soy/wheat
	Red River	wheat germ

Pasta

artichoke	semolina	spinach
buckwheat	soy	whole wheat
corn	spelt	quinoa

Breads

bran muffins	flatbread	rye
buckwheat	gluten-free	soy loaf
corn muffins	multi-grain	sprouted wheat
crispbread	rice cakes	whole wheat
essene	spelt	

Nuts and Seeds

almonds	peanuts	pumpkin seeds
brazil	pecans	sesame seeds
cashews	pinenuts	sunflower seeds
chestnuts (occasionally)	pistachios	walnuts
hazelnuts		

Nut and Seed Butters

almond   tahini

Spices and Condiments

apple cider vinegar	honey	rosemary
basil	kelp powder	scallions
bay leaf	maple syrup	sea salt
cayenne	miso	tamari
chervil	nutri or engivita yeast	tarragon
cloves	onion	thyme
dill	oregano	vegetable salt
dry mustard	parsley	
garlic	pure vanilla	

Oils

All oils should be cold pressed.

canola	peanut	soy
grape	safflower	sunflower
olive	sesame	

Herbal Teas

alfalfa	golden seal	peppermint
chamomile	parsley	rose hip
dandelion	ging seng	

Tofu

1/2 – 1 square per day

■　　■　　　■

Menus for Type O

SUNDAY	MONDAY	TUESDAY
Breakfast *water with lemon* *½ grapefruit* *1 poached egg* *1 or 2 slices whole-wheat toast* *1 cup herbal tea*	*Breakfast* *water with lemon* *½ grapefruit* *whole grain cereal* *1 cup herbal tea*	*Breakfast* *water with lemon* *½ grapefruit* *1 or 2 poached eggs* *1 cup herbal tea*
Lunch *Lettuce,* *beansprouts,* *chicory, celery* *¼ square tofu* *Dressing:* *Safflower oil/* *lemon juice* *1 cup herbal tea* *rice cakes or 1 slice* *whole grain cereal*	*Lunch* *tomato, lettuce,* *tofu, vegetables* *1 slice whole-wheat toast* *1 cup herbal tea*	*Lunch* *Wedges of lettuce,* *green vegetables,* *tofu, sprouts,* *1 cup herbal tea*
Dinner *¼ lb. steak,* *lean, broiled* *Salad:* *Cucumbers and* *beansprouts, peas* *Dressing:* *Safflower/* *lemon juice* *Vegetables:* *Steamed* *Kale,* *Swiss chard,* *broccoli,* *dandelion* *Beverage:* *1 cup herbal tea*	*Dinner* *2 lean lamb* *chops, or pasta* *Salad:* *Lettuce,* *beansprouts,* *chicory, tofu* *Dressing:* *Safflower oil/* *lemon juice* *Beverage:* *1 cup herbal tea*	*Dinner* *¼ chicken, skin* *removed,* *broiled, baked,* *boiled* *Vegetables:* *Steamed* *broccoli, asparagus,* *string beans, peas* *Salad:* *Lettuce, cucumbers,* *sprouts, tofu* *Dressing:* *Safflower oil/* *lemon juice* *Beverage:* *1 cup herbal tea*

Late night snack: either 1 apple or ½ grapefruit. When eating fruit before a meal, always wait ten minutes before eating the rest of the food.

WEDNESDAY	THURSDAY	FRIDAY	SATURDAY
Breakfast water with lemon ½ grapefruit whole grain cereal 1 cup herbal tea	*Breakfast* water with lemon ½ grapefruit 1 or 2 slices whole- wheat bread toasted 1 cup herbal tea	*Breakfast* ½ grapefruit 1 or 2 slices whole- wheat bread toasted 1 cup herbal tea	*Breakfast* ½ grapefruit whole grain cereal 1 cup herbal tea
Lunch Lettuce, sprouts, vegetables, tofu 1 cup herbal tea	*Lunch* Wedges of lettuce, tofu, vegetables, sprouts 1 cup herbal tea	*Lunch* 8 oz. plain yogurt with 2 tbsp. wheat- germ 1 cup herbal tea	*Lunch* Salad: Lettuce, cucumbers, beansprouts, tomato, brown rice with tofu Dressing: Safflower oil/ lemon juice 1 cup herbal tea
Dinner Salmon steak baked/broiled Salad: Watercress, tomato, mush- rooms, chicory, celery, kale, beansprouts Dressing: Safflower/ lemon Beverage: 1 cup herbal tea	*Dinner* 1 veal chop, lean, broiled Salad: Spinach with mushrooms Dressing: Safflower/ lemon Vegetables: Steamed beet leaves, dandelion, asparagus Beverage: 1 cup herbal tea	*Dinner* 1 flounder fillet baked/broiled Salad: Lettuce, cucum- bers, bean- sprouts, ¼ square tofu Dressing: Safflower/ lemon Vegetables: Steamed broccoli Beverage: 1 cup herbal tea	*Dinner* ½ chicken, skin removed, baked, boiled, broiled Salad: Lettuce, celery, cucumbers, beansprouts Dressing: Safflower/lemon Vegetables: Steamed spin- ach, escarole, broccoli, kale Beverage: 1 cup herbal tea

 # Type A Menu

The Type A should not eat meat, dairy products, or whole-wheat products. This diet is often too rigorous in the beginning. Thus it is often wise to eat fish, chicken, or turkey two to three days a week while becoming accustomed to such a menu. Interestingly, most Type A's find the vegetarian diet suits them and are quite comfortable following it.

_ Milk and Milk Products_

soybean milk

Vegetables

agar
all lettuces
artichokes
asparagus
avocado
bamboo sprouts
bean sprouts
beets
beet greens
boiled carrots
broccoli
celery
chicory
cucumber
daikon
dandelion greens

endive
escarole
fennel
green pepper
kale
kohlrabi
lentils (once a month)
lima beans
mushrooms
okra
olives
peas
parsley
pumpkin
radishes

red pepper
rugola
seaweed
shallots
spinach (once a month)
squash (all types)
Swiss chard
sweet potato
tomatoes
water chestnuts
watercress
white corn
white potato
zucchini

Fruits

apricots
Bing cherries
black grapes
blueberries
cantaloupe

coconut
cranberries
currants
custard fruit
dates

elderberries
figs (fresh)
gooseberries
grapefruit
guava

Fruits

kiwi	papaya	pomegranate
lemons	peaches	raisins
lime	pears	raspberries
loganberries	persimmons	rhubarb (occasionally)
mangoes	pineapple	strawberries
oranges (occasionally)	plums (dark Italian)	watermelon

Fruit Juices

apricot	cranberry	grapefruit
blueberry	diluted papaya	water and lemon
cherry	grape	

Grains and Cereals

brown rice	corn germ	soy flakes
bulgur	cornmeal	soy granules
corn bran	rolled oats	

Pasta

artichoke	rice noodle	vermicelle
corn	soya	

Breads

corn muffins	gluten-free	rye (occasionally)
essene	rice cakes	soy loafs
flatbread	rye crisp	sprouted wheat

Nuts and Seeds

almonds	pecans	pumpkin seeds
brazil	pinenuts	sesame seeds
chestnut (occasionally)	pistachios	sunflower seeds
filberts		

___ Nut and Seed Butters ___

almond   peanut (if fresh)   tahini

__ Spices and Condiments __

agar	dulse flakes	parsley
basil	garlic	rosemary
bay leaf	honey	scallion
cayenne	kelp powder	sea salt
chives	maple syrup	tarragon
cinnamon	miso	thyme
cloves	nutmeg	vegetable salt
dill	oregano	wheat-free tamari
dry mustard		

_____ Oils _____

All oils should be cold pressed.

olive   sesame   sunflower
safflower   soy

_____ Herbal Teas _____

alfalfa   dandelion   peppermint
chamomile

_____ Tofu _____

1/2 – 2 squares per day

■   ■   ■

Menus for Type A

SUNDAY	MONDAY	TUESDAY
Breakfast *water with lemon* *1 or 2 slices toasted* *soya bread with tofu spread* *1 cup herbal tea*	*Breakfast* *water with lemon* *cereal* *1 cup herbal tea*	*Breakfast* *water with lemon* *1 or 2 slices toasted* *soya bread* *1 cup herbal tea*
Lunch *Salad:* *Lettuce,* *tomato, celery,* *watercress,* *cucumber,* *beansprouts* *brown rice* *1 slice toasted soya bread* *Dressing:* *Safflower oil* *Lemon juice* *Beverage:* *1 cup herbal tea*	*Lunch* *Salad:* *Lettuce, stalk of* *celery, one* *tomato, ½* *square tofu,* *parsley* *brown rice* *Dressing:* *Safflower oil* *Lemon juice* *Beverage:* *1 cup herbal tea*	*Lunch* *Salad:* *Sections of 1* *grapefruit and 1* *orange on a bed* *of lettuce* *Beverage:* *1 cup herbal tea*
Dinner *¼ chicken, skin* *removed,* *boiled or* *broiled* *Vegetables* *(steamed only):* *Swiss chard,* *dandelion,* *asparagus* *Salad:* *Lettuce, cucum-* *ber, celery,* *beansprouts,* *tomato* *½ square tofu* *Dressing:* *Safflower oil* *Lemon juice* *Beverage:* *1 cup herbal tea*	*Dinner* *1 salmon steak* *broiled* *Vegetables* *(steamed only):* *Kale, string* *beans, broccoli* *tips* *Salad:* *Lettuce,* *tomato, sprouts* *Dressing:* *Safflower oil* *Lemon juice* *Beverage:* *1 cup herbal tea*	*Dinner* *¼ chicken, skin* *removed,* *boiled or* *broiled* *Vegetables* *(steamed only):* *Dandelion,* *broccoli tips,* *asparagus* *Salad:* *Lettuce, cucum-* *ber, celery, par-* *sley* *Dressing:* *Safflower oil* *Lemon juice* *Beverage:* *1 cup herbal tea*

When eating fruit before a meal, always wait ten minutes before eating the rest of the food.

WEDNESDAY	THURSDAY	FRIDAY	SATURDAY
Breakfast *water with lemon* *1 or 2 slices* *toasted soya bread* *1 cup herbal tea*	*Breakfast* *water with lemon* *1 or 2 slices* *toasted soya bread* *1 cup herbal tea*	*Breakfast* *water with lemon* *1 or 2 slices* *toasted soya bread* *1 cup herbal tea*	*Breakfast* *water with lemon* *1 or 2 slices toasted* *with tofu spread* *1 cup herbal tea*
Lunch *Salad:* *mixed lettuces* *1 can of water-* *packed sardines* *Vegetables* *Beverage:* *1 cup herbal tea*	*Lunch* *Salad:* *Lettuce* *Dressing:* *Safflower oil* *Lemon juice* *2 eggs poached* *Beverage:* *1 cup herbal tea*	*Lunch* *Salad:* *Lettuce, cucum-* *bers, water-* *cress,* *beansprouts,* *celery, tomato,* *½ square tofu,* *parsley* *Dressing:* *Safflower oil* *Lemon juice* *Beverage:* *1 cup herbal tea*	*Lunch* *Salad:* *Sections of 1* *grapefruit and 1* *orange on a bed* *of lettuce* *1 slice toasted* *soya bread* *Beverage:* *1 cup herbal tea*
Dinner *½ grapefruit* *Salad:* *Lettuce, celery,* *tomato, cucum-* *ber, parsley,* *spinach,* *chicory, raw* *fresh mush-* *rooms* *½ square tofu* *1 or 2 slices of* *soya bread* *Dressing:* *Safflower oil* *Lemon juice* *Beverage:* *1 cup herbal tea*	*Dinner* *½ lb. flounder,* *broiled* *Vegetables* *(steamed only):* *String beans* *Salad:* *Lettuce,* *beansprouts,* *celery,* *cucumbers* *Dressing:* *Safflower oil* *Lemon juice* *Beverage:* *1 cup herbal tea*	*Dinner* *Vegetables* *(steamed only):* *Kale, kelp,* *okra, Swiss* *chard, snow-* *pea pods* *Salad:* *Lettuce, celery,* *chicory, water-* *cress,* *beansprouts,* *parsley,* *brown rice* *Dressing:* *Safflower oil* *Lemon juice* *1 slice soya toast* *Beverage:* *1 cup herbal tea*	*Dinner* *½ lb. haddock* *Salad:* *Lettuce, tomato,* *chicory, celery,* *beansprouts,* *cucumber, parsley* *Dressing:* *Safflower oil* *Lemon juice* *Beverage:* *1 cup herbal tea* *Steamed vegetables*

  *Type B Menu*

Type B shares the dietary requirements of O and A. The key is moderation. He can choose from a broad range of vegetarian and animal-protein foods.

Meats
three servings per week

beef (1 or 2x month)	duck	turkey
calf's liver	internal organs	veal
(occasionally)	lamb	venison
chicken	pheasant	

Fish
two servings per week

bass	halibut	sea bass
bluefish	herring	sea trout
brook trout	mai mai	scrod
cod	orange roughy	skate
flounder	pickerel	sole
grouper	pike	turbot
haddock	red snapper	whiting
	salmon	white snapper

Eggs
three to four per week (boiled or poached)

Cheese

Brie (occasionally)	goat	quark
cottage	gouda	ricotta
Edam	Gruyère	Swiss
farmer's	mozzarella	

_ Milk and Milk Products _
two servings per week except soybean milk which may be taken as desired

buttermilk
goat's milk
rice milk

skim milk
soybean milk

sweet butter
yogurt

_____ Whole Grains _____

barley
brown rice
buckwheat

kamut
kasha
millet

pasta
pilaf
spelt
wheat grains

_____ Vegetables _____

agar
alfalfa
artichokes
asparagus
bamboo sprouts
bean sprouts
beans (all types)
beets
beet greens
boiled carrots
broccoli
brussels sprouts
(once a month)
celery
chicory
collards
cucumber
daikon
dandelion greens
eggplant

endive
escarole
fresh peas
fiddleheads
green pepper
green onions
kale
kelp
kohlrabi
leeks
lentils (occasionally)
lettuce (all kinds)
mushrooms
mustard greens
(occasionally)
okra
olives
parsley
spinach (once a month)

pumpkin
radishes (occasionally)
raw carrots (occasionally)
red cabbage
red pepper
rugola
seaweed
snow-pea pods
squash (all types)
Swiss chard
sweet potato
tomatoes (once a month)
turnips (occasionally)
watercress
water chestnuts
white cabbage
(occasionally)
white potato
zucchini (once a week)

Fruits

apple (occasionally)
apricots
Bing cherries
blackberries
blueberries
cantaloupe
coconut
cranberries
currants
dates
elderberry
figs

gooseberries
grapefruit
grapes (all kinds)
guava
honeydew
kiwi
lemons
limes
loganberries
mangoes
muskmelon
oranges (occasionally)

papaya
peaches
pear (once a week)
pineapple
plums (dark Italian)
pomegranate
raisins
raspberries
tangerines
strawberries
watermelon

Fruit Juices

apple (once or
twice a week)
apricot
blueberry

cherry
cranberry
grape
grapefruit

orange
papaya
water and lemon

Cereals

bran*
cornmeal[†]
cream of whole wheat*
Familia*
5-grain*

Grapenuts*
oatmeal*
puffed rice[†]
millet*
Red River*

shredded wheat*
soya/wheat[†]
soy flakes[†]
soy granules[†]
spelt
wheatgerm*

4 servings per week   *† 3 servings per week*

Breads

bran muffins*
buckwheat*
corn muffins
essene
flatbread

gluten-free
multi-grain*
rye
rice cakes

rye crisps*
soy loafs
spelt
sprouted wheat
whole wheat*

3 servings per week

_____ Nuts and Seeds _____

almonds	pecans	sesame seeds
brazil	pinenuts	sunflower seeds
chestnuts (occasionally)	pistachios	walnuts
hazelnuts	pumpkin seeds	

___ Nut and Seed Butters ___

almond   tahini

__ Spices and Condiments __

apple cider vinegar	honey	pure vanilla
basil	kelp powder	rosemary
bay leaf	maple syrup	scallions
cayenne	miso	sea salt
chervil	nutri or engivita yeast	tamari
cloves	onion	tarragon
dill	oregano	thyme
dry mustard	parsley	vegetable salt
garlic		

_____ Oils _____

All oils should be cold pressed.

canola	olive	sesame
grape	peanut	soy
	safflower	sunflower

_____ Herbal Teas _____

alfalfa	ging seng	parsley
chamomile	golden seal	peppermint
dandelion	green tea	rose hip (occasionally)

_____ Tofu _____

1/2 – 2 squares per day

■

Menus for Type B

SUNDAY	MONDAY	TUESDAY
Breakfast water with lemon ½ grapefruit 1 or 2 slices toasted soya bread tofu spread 1 cup herbal tea	*Breakfast* water with lemon ½ grapefruit cereal 1 cup herbal tea	*Breakfast* water with lemon ½ grapefruit 1 or 2 slices toasted whole-wheat bread tofu spread 1 cup herbal tea
Lunch ½ grapefruit 1 orange 1 apple grapes, mangos, made into a fruit salad	*Lunch* Salad: Lettuce, tomato, beansprouts, celery, cucum- ber, chicory, parsley, brown rice Dressing: Safflower oil/lemon ½ square tofu 1 slice soya bread toasted Beverage: 1 cup herbal tea	*Lunch* ½ grapefruit 1 orange on bed of lettuce 1 slice whole- wheat bread toasted tofu spread Beverage: 1 cup herbal tea
Dinner ½ chicken, skin removed, broiled, baked or boiled Vegetables: Steamed beet leaves, broccoli, kale Salad: Cucumbers Dressing: Safflower oil/ lemon Beverage: 1 cup herbal tea	*Dinner* 1 salmon steak baked Salad: Lettuce, cucum- bers, chicory, beansprouts Dressing: Safflower oil/ lemon Vegetables: Steamed string beans, dan- delion, broccoli tips Beverage: 1 cup herbal tea	*Dinner* ¼ chicken, skin removed, broiled Vegetables (steamed): Beet leaves, dandelion, asparagus Salad: Lettuce, bean- sprouts, cucum- bers Dressing: Safflower/ lemon Beverage: 1 cup herbal tea

When eating fruit before a meal, always wait ten minutes before you continue eating the rest of the food.

WEDNESDAY	THURSDAY	FRIDAY	SATURDAY
Breakfast	*Breakfast*	*Breakfast*	*Breakfast*
water with lemon	water with lemon	water with lemon	water with lemon
½ grapefruit	½ grapefruit	½ grapefruit	½ grapefruit
cereal	1 or 2 slices toasted	1 slice toasted	1 or 2 eggs
1 cup herbal tea	whole-wheat bread	soya bread	1 cup herbal tea
	tofu spread	1 cup herbal tea	
	1 cup herbal tea		
Lunch	*Lunch*	*Lunch*	*Lunch*
½ cantaloupe	2 hard-boiled	Salad:	Spinach salad
watermelon	eggs	Lettuce wedges	with fresh
kiwi slices	Lettuce, vegetables	⅛ square tofu spread	mushrooms
1 cup herbal tea	Beverage:	1 or 2 slices toasted	brown rice
	1 cup herbal tea	soya bread	⅛ square tofu
		Beverage:	Dressing:
		1 cup herbal tea	Safflower oil/
			lemon
			Beverage:
			1 cup herbal tea
Dinner	*Dinner*	*Dinner*	*Dinner*
Salad:	1 halibut steak	½ chicken, skin	¼ - ½ lb. veal,
Spinach, beet	Vegetables:	removed,	or beef, lean,
leaves, lettuce,	Steamed kale,	broiled	broiled
chicory, mush-	escarole	Vegetables:	Vegetables:
rooms, tomato,	Salad:	Steamed broc-	Steamed kale,
beansprouts	Lettuce, cucum-	coli, asparagus	asparagus
½ square tofu	bers	Salad:	Salad:
Vegetables	Dressing:	Lettuce, ½	Lettuce, tomato,
(steamed):	Safflower oil/	tomato, cucum-	celery, water-
brown rice	lemon	bers,	cress,
Asparagus,	Beverage:	beansprouts	beansprouts
broccoli	1 cup herbal tea	Dressing:	Dressing:
Dressing:		Safflower oil/	Safflower oil/
Safflower oil/lemon		lemon	lemon
Beverage:		Beverage:	Beverage:
1 cup herbal tea		1 cup herbal tea	1 cup herbal tea

Night snack: Apple once a week. Remainder of days ½ grapefruit.

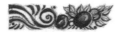 ## Type AB Menu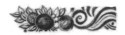

The Type AB should, for the most part, not eat meat, dairy products, or whole-wheat products. One serving or 2 of chicken per week is allowed.

Fish

two to three servings per week

cod	mai mai	sea bass
flounder	orange roughy	sea trout
haddock	salmon	shad
halibut	scrod	sole

Milk and Milk Products

soybean milk
rice milk

Vegetables

agar	dandelion greens	radishes
all lettuces	endive	red pepper
artichokes	escarole	rugola
asparagus	fennel	seaweed
avocado	green pepper	shallots
bamboo sprouts	kale	spinach (once a month)
bean sprouts	kohlrabi	squash (all types)
beet greens	lentils (once a month)	sweet potato
beets	lima beans	Swiss chard
boiled carrots	mushrooms	tomatoes
broccoli	okra	water chestnuts
celery	olives	watercress
chicory	parsley	white corn
cucumber	peas	white potato
daikon	pumpkin	zucchini

Fruits

apricots	figs (fresh)	peaches
black grapes	gooseberries	pears
Bing cherries	grapefruit	persimmons
blueberries	guava	pineapple
cantaloupe	kiwi	plums (dark Italian)
coconut	lemons	pomegranate
cranberries	limes	raisins
currants	loganberries	raspberries
custard fruit	mangoes	rhubarb (occasionally)
dates	oranges (occasionally)	strawberries
elderberries	papaya	watermelon

Fruit Juices

apricot	cranberry	grapefruit
blueberry	diluted papaya	water and lemon
cherry	grape	

Grains and Cereals

brown rice	cornmeal	soy flakes
bulgur	oat bran	soy granules
corn bran	rice bran	spelt
corn germ	rolled oats	sprouted wheat

Pasta

artichoke	rice noodle	vermicelle
corn	soya	spelt

Breads

corn muffins	gluten-free	rye crisp
essene	rice cakes	soy loafs
flatbread	rye (occasionally)	sprouted wheat
spelt	kamut	

_____ Nuts and Seeds _____

almonds	pecans	sesame seeds
brazil	pinenuts	sunflower seeds
chestnut (occasionally)	pistachios	walnuts
filberts	pumpkin seeds	

___ Nut and Seed Butters ___

almond	peanut (if fresh) (very occasionally)	tahini

__ Spices and Condiments__

agar	dulse flakes	parsley
basil	garlic	rosemary
bay leaf	honey	scallion
cayenne	kelp powder	tarragon
chives	maple syrup	thyme
cinnamon	miso	vegetable salt
cloves	nutmeg	wheat-free tamari
dill	oregano	
dry mustard		

_____ Oils _____

All oils should be cold pressed.

olive	sesame	sunflower
safflower	soy	canola
		grape

_____ Herbal Teas _____

alfalfa	dandelion	rose hip (occasionally)
chamomile	peppermint	

_____ Tofu _____

2 squares per day all types

■

 ## Menus for Type AB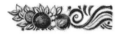

A Type AB person should start with the same meals as Type A. Slowly, small amounts of other foods — chicken, fish, whole-wheat products, skim milk and cheese — can be added. By monitoring the response to these additions, the right levels can be determined. If, for example, nasal congestion develops after adding milk, the level is too high.

Type Oa Menu

This individual may have a wheat allergy. If you are a Type O, it is possible that you have A traits. If you suffer from allergies, you may consider giving up all dairy products except soybean milk. If this gives no relief, delete wheat products as well.

Meats

two servings per week

beef	duck	lungs
brain	heart	pheasant
buffalo	intestines	turkey
calf's liver	kidney	veal
chicken	lamb	venison

Fish

five servings per week

bass	halibut	scrod
bluefish	herring	sea bass
brook trout	mai mai	sea trout
cod	orange roughy	skate
flounder	pickerel	sole
grouper	pike	turbot
haddock	red snapper	white snapper
	salmon	whiting

Eggs

four to five per week, boiled or poached

Cheese

Brie	farmer's	Munster
Camembert	goat	neufachtel
cheddar	gouda	provolone
colby	Gruyère	quark low-fat
cottage	havarti	ricotta
Edam	mozzarella	Swiss

Milk and Milk Products

buttermilk	raw cow's milk	tiger's milk
goat's milk	skim	2%
institute spread*	soybean milk	yogurt
		rice

*Recipe for Institute Spread: 1/4 lb. sweet butter }
1/4 c. safflower oil } blend and
1 Vitamin E capsule } refrigerate
1 lethicin capsule }

Whole Grains

barley	kamut	pasta
brown rice	kasha	pilaf
buckwheat	millet	spelt
		wheat grains

Vegetables

agar	beet greens	daikon
alfalfa	beets	dandelion greens
artichokes	broccoli	eggplant
asparagus	carrots	endive
avocado	celery	escarole
bamboo sprouts	chicory	fennel
beans (all types)	chick peas	fresh peas
bean sprouts	cucumber	green rhubarb
kale	okra	Swiss chard

Vegetables

kelp	olives	tomatoes
kohlrabi	onions	water chestnuts
leeks	seaweed	watercress
lentils	savoy cabbage	white cabbage
lettuce (all types)	snow-pea pods	white corn
mushrooms	spinach (once a month)	yeast
mustard greens	squash (all types)	yellow corn

Fruits

apples (occasionally)	elderberries	pears
apricots	figs	persimmons
bananas (once a month)	grapefruit	pineapple
blackberries	guava	plums (dark Italian)
black grapes	honeydew melons	pomegranate
blueberries	kiwi	raisins
cantaloupe	lemons	raspberries
cherries (all kinds)	limes	star apple
coconut	mangoes	strawberries
currants (occasionally)	oranges	tangerines
custard fruit	papaya	watermelon
dates	peaches	

Fruit Juices

apple	cherry	orange
apricot	cranberry	papaya
blueberry	grape	water and lemon
carrot (occasionally)	grapefruit	

Cereals

bran	millet	shredded wheat
cornmeal	oatmeal	soya/wheat
cream of whole wheat	puffed rice	soy flakes
Familia	quinoa	soy granules
5-grain	Red River	spelt
Grapenuts		wheat germ

Pasta

artichoke	semolina	spinach
buckwheat	soy	whole wheat
corn		spelt

Breads

bran muffins	flatbread	rye
buckwheat	gluten-free	soy loaf
corn muffins	multi-grain	spelt
crispbread	rice cakes	sprouted wheat
essene		whole wheat

Nuts and Seeds

almonds	peanuts	pumpkinseeds
brazil	pecans	sesame seeds
cashews	pinenuts	sunflower seeds
chestnuts	pistachios	walnuts
hazelnuts		

Nut and Seed Butters

almond	tahini

Spices and Condiments

apple cider vinegar	honey	rosemary
basil	kelp powder	scallions
bay leaf	maple syrup	sea salt
cayenne	miso	tamari
chervil	nutri or engivita yeast	tarragon
cloves	onion	thyme
dill	oregano	vegetable salt
dry mustard	parsley	
garlic	pure vanilla	

Oils

All oils should be cold pressed.

olive	safflower	soy
peanut	sesame	sunflower
	grape	canola

Herbal Teas

alfalfa	dandelion	parsley
chamomile	ging seng	peppermint
chick weed	golden seal	rose hip

Tofu

as much as desired

■

Type Ob Menu

Meat

four servings per week

beef	duck	lungs
brain	heart	pheasant
buffalo	intestines	turkey
calf's liver	kidney	veal
chicken	lamb	venison

Fish

three servings per week

bass	halibut	scrod
bluefish	herring	sea bass
brook trout	mai mai	sea trout
cod	orange roughy	skate
flounder	pickerel	sole
grouper	pike	turbot
haddock	red snapper	white snapper
	salmon	whiting

Eggs

four to five per week, boiled or poached

Cheese

two servings per week

Brie	farmer's	Munster
Camembert	goat	neufachtel
cheddar	gouda	provolone
colby	Gruyère	quark low-fat
cottage	havarti	ricotta
Edam	mozzarella	Swiss

Milk and Milk Products

buttermilk	raw cow's milk	tiger's milk
goat's milk	skim	2%
institute spread*	soybean milk	yogurt

*Recipe for Institute Spread: 1/4 lb. sweet butter }
1/4 c. safflower oil } blend and
1 Vitamin E capsule } refrigerate
1 lethicin capsule }

Whole Grains

barley	kasha	pilaf
brown rice	millet	wheat grains
buckwheat	pasta	

Vegetables

agar	beet greens	daikon
alfalfa	beets	dandelion greens
artichokes	broccoli	eggplant
asparagus	carrots	endive
avocado	celery	escarole
bamboo sprouts	chicory	fennel
bean sprouts	chick peas	fresh peas
beans (all types)	cucumber	green rhubarb

Vegetables

kale
kelp
kohlrabi
leeks
lentils
lettuce (all types)
mushrooms
mustard greens

okra
olives
onions
seaweed
savoy cabbage
snow-pea pods
spinach (once a month)
squash (all types)

Swiss chard
tomatoes
water chestnuts
watercress
white cabbage
white corn
yeast
yellow corn

Fruits

apples
apricots
bananas (once a month)
blackberries
black grapes
blueberries
cantaloupe
cherries (all kinds)
coconut
currants (occasionally)
custard fruit
dates

elderberries
figs
grapefruit
guava
honeydew melons
kiwi
lemons
limes
mangoes
oranges
papaya
peaches

pears
persimmons
pineapple
plums (dark Italian)
pomegranate
raisins
raspberries
star apples
strawberries
tangerines
watermelon

Fruit Juices

apple
apricot
blueberry
carrot (occasionally)

cherry
cranberry
grape
grapefruit

papaya
orange
water and lemon

Cereals

bran
cornmeal
cream of whole wheat
Familia
5-grain

grapenuts
millet
oatmeal
puffed rice
Red River

shredded wheat
soya/wheat
soy flakes
soy granules
wheat germ

Pasta

artichoke	semolina	spinach
buckwheat	soy	whole wheat
corn		

Breads

bran muffins	flatbread	rye
buckwheat	gluten-free	soy loaf
corn muffins	multi-grain	sprouted wheat
crispbread	rice cakes	whole wheat
essene		

Nuts and Seeds

almonds	peanuts	sesame seeds
brazil	pecans	sunflower seeds
cashews	pinenuts	walnuts
chestnuts	pistachios	
hazelnuts	pumpkinseeds	

Nut and Seed Butters

almond   tahini

Spices and Condiments

apple cider vinegar	honey	pure vanilla
basil	kelp powder	rosemary
bay leaf	maple syrup	scallions
cayenne	miso	sea salt
chervil	nutri or engivita yeast	tamari
cloves	onion	tarragon
dill	oregano	thyme
dry mustard	parsley	vegetable salt
garlic		

Oils

All oils should be cold pressed.

olive	safflower	soy
peanut	sesame	sunflower

Herbal Teas

alfalfa	golden seal	peppermint
chamomile	parsley	rose hip
dandelion		

Tofu

1/2 square per day

■

Type Ao Menu

Meat

one serving per week

brain	heart	lungs
calf's liver	intestines	pheasant
chicken	kidney	turkey
duck	lamb	

Fish

one serving per week

bass	halibut	scrod
bluefish	herring	sea bass
brook trout	mai mai	sea trout
cod	orange roughy	skate
flounder	pickerel	sole
grouper	pike	turbot
haddock	red snapper	white snapper
	salmon	whiting

Eggs
three per week, boiled, or poached

Cheese
if any 1x each month

cottage
farmer's

mozzarella

ricotta

Milk and Milk Products

rice milk

soybean milk

Vegetables

agar	dandelion greens	radishes
all lettuces	endive	red pepper
artichokes	escarole	rugola
asparagus	fennel	seaweed
avocado	green pepper	shallots
bamboo sprouts	kale	spinach (once a month)
bean sprouts	kohlrabi	squash (all types)
beet greens	lentils (once a month)	sweet potato
beets	lima beans	Swiss chard
boiled carrots	mushrooms	tomatoes
broccoli	okra	water chestnuts
celery	olives	watercress
chicory	parsley	white corn
cucumber	peas	white potato
daikon	pumpkin	zucchini

Fruits

apricots	cranberry	gooseberries
Bing cherries	currants	grapefruit
black grapes	custard fruit	guava
blueberries	dates	kiwi
cantaloupe	elderberries	lemons
coconut	figs (fresh)	limes

Fruits

loganberries	persimmons	raspberries
mangoes	pineapple	rhubarb (occasionally)
oranges (occasionally)	plums (dark Italian)	strawberries
papaya	pomegranate	tangerines
peaches	raisins	watermelon
pears		

Fruit Juices

apricot	cranberry	grapefruit
blueberry	diluted papaya	water and lemon
cherry	grape	

Grains and Cereals

brown rice	millet	soy flakes
bulgur	oat bran	soy granules
corn bran	puffed rice	whole wheat
corn germ	rolled oats	(occasionally)
corn meal		

Pasta

artichoke	rice noodle	spelt
corn	soya	vermicelle

Breads

corn muffins	gluten-free	rye crisp
essene	rice cakes	soy loaf
flatbread	rye (occasionally)	spelt
		sprouted wheat

Nuts and Seeds

almonds	pecans	sesame seeds
brazil	pinenuts	sunflower seeds
chestnuts (occasionally)	pistachios	walnuts
filberts	pumpkin seeds	

___ Nut and Seed Butters ___

almond	peanut (if fresh)	tahini

__ Spices and Condiments __

agar	dulse flakes	parsley
basil	garlic	rosemary
bay leaf	honey	scallion
cayenne	kelp powder	sea salt
chives	maple syrup	tarragon
cinnamon	miso	thyme
cloves	nutmeg	vegetable salt
dill	oregano	wheat-free tamari
dry mustard		

_____ Oils _____

All oils should be cold pressed.

canola	olive	soy
grape	safflower	sunflower
	sesame	

_____ Herbal Teas _____

alfalfa	dandelion	peppermint
chamomile		

_____ Tofu _____

1 – 2 squares per day

■

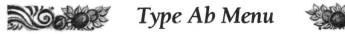 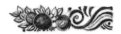

Type Ab Menu

Meat

one serving per week

brain	heart	lungs
calf's liver	intestines	pheasant
chicken	kidney	turkey
duck		

Fish

one serving per week

bass	herring	shad
bluefish	mai mai	sea bass
brook trout	orange roughy	sea trout
cod	pickerel	skate
flounder	pike	sole
grouper	red snapper	turbot
haddock	salmon	whiting
halibut	scrod	white snapper

Eggs

one per week, boiled or poached

Milk and Milk Products

soybean milk

Vegetables

agar	avocado	beets
all lettuces	bamboo sprouts	boiled carrots
artichokes	bean sprouts	broccoli
asparagus	beet greens	celery

Vegetables

chicory
cucumber
daikon
dandelion greens
endive
escarole
fennel
green pepper
kale
kohlrabi
lentils (once a month)

lima beans
mushrooms
okra
olives
parsley
peas
pumpkin
radishes
red pepper
rugola
seaweed

shallots
spinach (once a month)
squash (all types)
sweet potato
Swiss chard
tomatoes
water chestnuts
watercress
white corn
white potato
zucchini

Fruits

apricots
Bing cherries
black grapes
blueberries
cantaloupe
coconut
cranberries
currants
custard fruit
dates
elderberries

figs (fresh)
gooseberries
grapefruit
guava
kiwi
lemons
limes
loganberries
mangoes
oranges (occasionally)
papaya

peaches
pears
persimmons
pineapple
plums (dark Italian)
pomegranate
raisins
raspberries
rhubarb (occasionally)
strawberries
watermelon

Fruit Juices

apricot
blueberry
cherry

cranberry
diluted papaya
grape

grapefruit
water and lemon

Grains and Cereals

brown rice
bulgur
corn bran
corn germ

cornmeal
millet
oat bran
puffed rice

rolled oats
soy flakes
soy granules
sprouted grain

Pasta

artichoke	rice noodle	vermicelle
corn	soya	

Breads

corn muffins	kamut	soy loaf
essene	rice cakes	spelt
flatbread	rye (occasionally)	sprouted wheat
gluten-free	rye crisp	

Nuts and Seeds

almonds	pecans	sesame seeds
brazil	pinenuts	sunflower seeds
chestnuts (occasionally)	pistachios	walnuts
filberts	pumpkin seeds	

Nut and Seed Butters

almond	peanut (if fresh)	tahini
	orc	

Spices and Condiments

agar	dulse flakes	parsley
basil	garlic	rosemary
bay leaf	honey	scallion
cayenne	kelp powder	sea salt
chives	maple syrup	tarragon
cinnamon	miso	thyme
cloves	nutmeg	vegetable salt
dill	oregano	wheat-free tamari
dry mustard		

Oils

All oils should be cold pressed.

canola	olive	soy
grape	safflower	sunflower
	sesame	

Herbal Teas

alfalfa   dandelion   peppermint
chamomile

Tofu

1-1/2 – 2 squares per day

◼

Type Bo Menu

Meat
five servings per week

beef (once a month)   internal organs   turkey
calf's liver (occasionally)   lamb   veal
chicken   pheasant   venison
duck

Fish
two servings per week

bass   herring   sea bass
bluefish   mai mai   sea trout
brook trout   orange roughy   skate
cod   pickerel   sole
flounder   pike   turbot
grouper   red snapper   white snapper
haddock   salmon   whiting
halibut   scrod

Eggs
three to four per week (boiled or poached)

Cheese

Brie (occasionally)
cottage
Edam
farmer's

goat
gouda
Gruyère
mozzarella

quark
ricotta
Swiss

Milk and Milk Products

buttermilk
goat's milk

rice
skim milk
soybean milk

sweet butter
yogurt

Whole Grains

barley
brown rice
buckwheat

kamut
kasha
millet

pasta
pilaf
spelt
wheat grains

Vegetables

agar
alfalfa
artichokes
asparagus
bamboo sprouts
bean sprouts
beans (all types)
beet greens
beets
boiled carrots
broccoli
brussels sprouts
(once a month)
celery
chicory
collards

cucumber
daikon
dandelion greens
eggplant
endive
escarole
fiddleheads
fresh peas
green onions
green pepper
kale
kelp
kohlrabi
leeks
lentils (occasionally)
lettuce (all kinds)

mushrooms
mustard greens
(occasionally)
okra
olives
parsley
pumpkin
radishes (occasionally)
raw carrots
(occasionally)
red cabbage
red pepper
rugola
seaweed
snow-pea pods
spinach (once a month)

Vegetables

squash (all types)
sweet potato
Swiss chard
tomatoes (once a month)

turnips (occasionally)
water chestnuts
watercress
white cabbage (occasionally)

white corn
white potato
zucchini (once a week)

Fruits

apples (occasionally)
apricots
Bing cherries
blueberries
blackberries
cantaloupe
coconut
cranberries
currants
dates
elderberry
figs

grapes (all kinds)
gooseberries
grapefruit
guava
honeydew
kiwi
lemons
limes
loganberries
mangoes
muskmelon
oranges (occasionally)

papaya
peaches
pear (once a week)
pineapple
plums (dark Italian)
pomegranate
raisins
raspberries
strawberries
tangerines
watermelon

Fruit Juices

apple (once or twice a week)
apricot
blueberry

cherry
cranberry
grape
grapefruit

orange
papaya
water and lemon

Cereals

bran*
cornmeal†
cream of whole wheat*
Familia*
5-grain*

Grapenuts*
millet*
oatmeal*
puffed rice†
Red River*

shredded wheat*
soy flakes†
soy granules†
soya/wheat†
wheat germ*

4 servings per week † 3 servings per week

Breads

bran muffins*	gluten-free	rye crisps*
buckwheat*	kamut	soy loafs
corn muffins	multi-grain*	spelt
essene	rice cakes	sprouted wheat
flatbread	rye	whole wheat*

* 3 servings per week

Nuts and Seeds

almonds	pecans	sesame seeds
brazil	pinenuts	sunflower seeds
chestnuts (occasionally)	pistachios	walnuts
hazelnuts	pumpkin seeds	

Nut and Seed Butters

almond   tahini

Spices and Condiments

apple cider vinegar	honey	pure vanilla
basil	kelp powder	rosemary
bay leaf	maple syrup	scallion
cayenne	miso	sea salt
chervil	nutri or engivita yeast	tamari
cloves	onion	tarragon
dill	oregano	thyme
dry mustard	parsley	vegetable salt
garlic		

Oils

All oils should be cold pressed.

canola	olive	sesame
grape	peanut	soy
	safflower	sunflower

Herbal Teas

alfalfa	dandelion	peppermint
chamomile	parsley	rose hip (occasionally)

Tofu

1 square per day

∎

Type Ba Menu

Meat

two servings per week

beef (once a month)	duck	turkey
calf's liver	internal organs	veal
(occasionally)	lamb	venison
chicken	pheasant	

Fish

three servings per week

bass	herring	sea bass
bluefish	mai mai	sea trout
brook trout	orange roughy	skate
cod	pickerel	sole
flounder	pike	turbot
grouper	red snapper	white snapper
haddock	salmon	whiting
halibut	scrod	

Eggs

three to four per week (boiled or poached)

Cheese

Brie (occasionally)	goat	quark
cottage	gouda	ricotta
Edam	Gruyère	Swiss
farmer's	mozzarella	

Milk and Milk Products

Two servings per week except soybean milk, which may be taken as desired. Those with allergies should eliminate dairy products (including all cheese), with the exception of soybean milk, altogether. Once allergies are eliminated, it may be possible to slowly re-introduce dairy products.

buttermilk	rice milk	sweet butter
goat's milk	skim milk	yogurt
	soybean milk	

Whole Grains

barley	kamut	pasta
brown rice	kasha	pilaf
buckwheat	millet	spelt
		wheat grains

Vegetables

agar	boiled carrots	dandelion greens
alfalfa	broccoli	eggplant
artichokes	brussels sprouts	endive
asparagus	(once a month)	escarole
bamboo sprouts	celery	fiddleheads
bean sprouts	chicory	fresh peas
beans (all types)	collards	green onions
beet greens	cucumber	green pepper
beets	daikon	kale

Vegetables

kelp
kohlrabi
leeks
lentils (occasionally)
lettuce (all kinds)
mushrooms
mustard greens
(occasionally)
okra
olives
parsley
pumpkin

radishes (occasionally)
raw carrots
(occasionally)
red cabbage
red pepper
rugola
seaweed
snow-pea pods
spinach (once a month)
squash (all types)
sweet potato

Swiss chard
tomatoes (once a
month)
turnips (occasionally)
water chestnuts
watercress
white cabbage
(occasionally)
white corn
white potato
zucchini

Fruits

apples (occasionally)
apricots
Bing cherries
blackberries
blueberries
cantaloupe
coconut
cranberries
currants
dates
elderberries
figs

gooseberries
grapes (all kinds)
grapefruit
guava
honeydew
kiwi
lemons
limes
loganberries
mangoes
muskmelon
oranges (occasionally)

papaya
peaches
pear (once a week)
pineapple
plums (dark Italian)
pomegranate
raisins
raspberries
strawberries
tangerines
watermelon

Fruit Juices

apple (once or
twice a week)
apricot
blueberry

cherry
cranberry
grape
grapefruit

orange
papaya
water and lemon

Cereals

bran*	Grapenuts*	shredded wheat*
cornmeal†	millet*	soy flakes†
cream of whole wheat*	oatmeal*	soy granules†
Familia*	puffed rice†	soya/wheat†
5-grain*	Red River*	wheat germ*

4 servings per week † 3 servings per week

Breads

bran muffins*	gluten-free	rye crisps*
buckwheat*	kamut	soy loaf
corn muffins	multi-grain*	spelt
essene	rice cakes	sprouted wheat
flatbread	rye	wholewheat*

3 servings per week

Nuts and Seeds

almonds	pecans	sesame seeds
brazil	pinenuts	sunflower seeds
chestnuts (occasionally)	pistachios	walnuts
hazelnuts	pumpkin seeds	

Nut and Seed Butters

almond   tahini

Spices and Condiments

apple cider vinegar	cayenne	dill
basil	chervil	dry mustard
bay leaf	cloves	garlic

Spices and Condiments

honey	oregano	sea salt
kelp powder	parsley	tamari
maple syrup	pure vanilla	tarragon
miso	rosemary	thyme
nutri or engivita yeast	scallion	vegetable salt
onion		

Oils

All oils should be cold pressed.

canola	olive	sesame
grape	peanut	soy
	safflower	sunflower

Herbal Teas

alfalfa	golden seal	rose hip (occasionally)
chamomile	parsley	slippery elm
dandelion	peppermint	

Tofu

1-1/2 – 2 squares per day

■

6

HOW TO
CREATE YOUR
OWN DIET

Few people can plunge straight into a new menu pattern. The changes are too great, and they are likely to give up after a few days or weeks. In this chapter, I show you how to modify your diet and lifestyle slowly, allowing your body and mind time to adjust to the new foods and patterns.

Type O

Level One

Eliminate processed and refined foods. Substitute whole-wheat products for breads made of white or enriched flour and do not eat processed cereals. Introduce whole-grain cereals, such as millet, oatmeal, cornmeal, and soy flakes, to replace sugared and puffed breakfast cereals.

Reduce beef and pork products. Select animal protein from veal, lamb, calf's liver, chicken, turkey, the internal organs of organically raised cattle (kidneys, heart, lungs), and fish. Eliminate commercially produced dairy products and choose milk, cheese, yogurt, and butter made from raw cows' milk or goats' milk.

Eliminate fried foods. Reduce alcohol consumption and cigarette smoking. Substitute honey for white or brown sugar.

Evaluate your physical exercise program. Your goal is to create a vigorous regimen appropriate to your age and physical condition. An hour or two of exercise such as jogging, swimming, bicycling, or gymnastics every day will greatly benefit you now.

Work into this step over a period of a month to a month-and-a-half.

Level Two

Animal protein should be eaten once a day every day. Choose one from the recommended selection in level five. Soft cheeses, including ricotta, farmer's, cottage, and mozzarella, may be eaten five times a week. A half a glass of whole milk may be drunk every day; and you can also have six eggs a week, and yogurt twice weekly.

You may eat whole-wheat products as often as you like, and you can also choose from such cereals as millet, oatmeal, cornmeal, soya/wheat, shredded wheat, wheat germ, and bran.

If you are younger than thirty, you may use butter made from raw cream, but in moderation. Type O's over thirty (the age at which your body's systems begin to slow and become more susceptible to the buildup of fatty deposits in your circulatory system) should switch to margarines made of such polyunsaturated oils as safflower, sunflower, or soy. Cold-pressed oils can be mixed with lemon or with apple cider vinegar and your choice of herbs for salad dressing.

Sea salt may be used in moderation; but kelp powder should be used sparingly because its rich iodine content may overstimulate your thyroid gland and increase your metabolic rate.

Vegetarian lunches should be introduced into your diet once or twice a week.

This step can be adapted over a period of two months. Once you have reached this stage successfully, there will be little change in your diet as you work toward level five, the ideal diet.

Level Three

Refer to level two for your allowed intake of animal protein.

Whole milk should now be reduced to four glasses a week, alternating with either skim or soy milk. (Regardless of the amount of cows' milk you drink, you may drink several glasses of soy milk a day.) Soft cheeses mentioned in level two may be eaten four times a week, yogurt twice a week. You should now lower your intake of eggs from six to four a week.

Lunches should now be vegetarian four to five times a week.

Olive oil should now be introduced in your diet. Take a tablespoon every other day to assist digestion and promote elimination.

Your physical regimen should now be fully created; to stimulate your body, take cold showers, hip baths, and saunas regularly.

Unless you are suffering with a serious illness, you can take three to four months to work into this program.

Level Four

Continue to follow the regimen outlined in level three with these changes: lunch (if it is not your main meal) should now be totally vegetarian; in addition, eat a square of tofu with every meal for additional protein.

Level Five

The ideal O diet is as follows: oatmeal, soya/wheat, cornmeal, millet, shredded wheat, wheat germ, or bran for breakfast with diluted skim milk or soy milk and a dab of honey. Bread may be selected from whole wheat or soy loafs.

Lunch, or the meal other than the main meal, should be entirely vegetarian, consisting of mixed salads and sprouts, with seeds or almonds. Tofu should be eaten four times a week, and you may eat soft cheeses four times a week, and yogurt twice a week. Four eggs are your weekly allowance.

The main meal of the day should be meat. The best balance is veal once a week, lamb, and calf's liver once every two weeks, chicken or turkey twice a week, internal organs (if available) once a week and fish the remaining nights. Remember, you must adapt your protein intake to your individual condition.

Type A

Level One

This is an evaluation step for those who are not yet following a dietary regimen and are still eating commercially processed foods. The average person with type-A blood will have a long journey to level five, with many foods to eliminate from his diet as he makes the adjustment to a vegetarian lifestyle. The A will have to be patient in altering his diet, but it is not impossible, nor even terribly difficult. I, myself, am an A, and a product of a good Italian family — which means that I had my share of pasta, sausages, and prosciutto to give up! Even though I had fond memories of spaghetti and clam sauce, when I decided to change my eating habits, it took only about six weeks to re-educate my taste buds and embrace a new way of eating. Take it from me: your palate quickly loses its hunger for certain tastes; it's your thoughts you must master. Control your thoughts and in a short period of time you can switch from, for example, scungilli to a fresh mixed salad without feeling deprived.

Before you try to eliminate meat and dairy products from your diet, first substitute better quality equivalents for the foods you are now eating. Substitute whole-grain breads and cereals, such as whole wheat, rye, rolled oats, and cornmeal, for products made with white flour and chemical additives. Canned foods should be replaced by fresh fruits and vegetables. Foods that have been preserved, flavored, or colored, or are chemically synthesized should be totally eliminated. Buy your own pure ingredients — bake your own cake, prepare your own pasta dinner, or steam your own whole, brown rice. Others have said it before, but there is no doubt about it: you are what you eat. So think about what you are putting into your body. Be aware when you are eating that food is fuel and a poor-grade fuel is going to clog and rob your human machine of its potential energy and efficiency. Try to control your cravings.

The same kind of descretion should apply when selecting meats. It is crucial to avoid all packed meats such as canned ham, frankfurters, and frozen fish. These products are usually preserved with salt and chemicals such as sodium nitrite, which has been linked with cancer. When shopping in the supermarket, be sure you buy only grade-A meats, with no additives. Meat should be well-sealed: exposure to air reduces its nutritional value. If you are now buying a lot of red meats, such as chopped beef, steaks, or roasts, or pork products, think about switching to veal, lamb, chicken, and turkey. The latter choices are leaner, have less uric acid, and smaller concentrations of steroids and antibiotics. Fish is also lean and is a purer food than meat or poultry.

Your main consideration in buying any food should be: is this substance in its purest, simplest state; as close as possible to the state in which the fruit fell from the tree, the vegetable grew from the earth, or the meat came from the animal?

Other factors that affect health and should now be examined are the amount of alcohol you drink, the number of cigarettes you smoke per day, and your current exercise program. Hard alcohol, which robs the body of many nutrients and debilitates the liver, should be eliminated and replaced by moderate quantities of red or white wine. Consider the harm cigarettes inflict on the entire body: they weaken the lungs, destroy Vitamin C, which can lower your resistance against disease, and have been proved to contain cancer-causing agents. If you really want to recover your health fully, try to cut down with the goal of eventually eliminating cigarette smoking.

Lastly, evaluate the amount of physical activity you are currently engaged in. It your occupation demanding? Do you exercise? How much? Are you exerting yourself? Remember the A should try to find peace through exercise and should not be stressing himself by attempting to be a marathon runner or a Charles Atlas.

The A should remain at this step for one to two months.

Level Two

At this level you will be concerned with narrowing your selection of foods. Your choice of meats should now only include veal, lamb, chicken, turkey, or fish. Beef and pork products should be completely eliminated. Whole-wheat products and wheat-derived grains that were introduced in level one should now be alternated with soy products. For instance, whole-wheat bread may be eaten three or four times a week, on the other days select a soy loaf. Soy beans, soy flakes or granules should be substituted for millet, cracked wheat, or buckwheat. A square of tofu should be eaten with every meal, too.

Dairy products should also be cut back. Milk should be diluted with water, soft cheese substituted for hard cheese, eggs reduced to four or five a week, and yogurt eaten only twice a week. Soy milk may be substituted for raw milk. Goats' milk products are better than raw milk, cheeses, and yogurt.

You should eat vegetables steamed, not raw, at this level. This will help the body adapt to these highly laxative foods and have a gentler effect on the bowels than raw vegetables. As your body adjusts to fresh foods, which may happen at this level or later in the program, you can eat your vegetables either steamed or raw.

Lunch should gradually become a vegetarian meal. If you are not ready to have raw salads as your meal, make a plate of steamed vegetables. If your body adapts readily to raw foods, then prepare a salad to your liking, but omit your favorite salad dressing. From this point on, use only oil and lemon and a few herbs such as rosemary, oregano, basil, or dill. Cider vinegar especially should be avoided as it is too acidic for your body. Sea salt should now be used instead of regular table salt. Kelp powder, which is beneficial to a hyperactive thyroid, may also be used as a condiment on salads, vegetables, or meat dishes.

Stay on this diet for about two months.

Level Three

All animal protein except chicken and fish should now be eliminated from your diet. It is also recommend that you reduce your intake of animal protein and eat chicken and fish only twice a week. Your selection of fish should include: bluefish, salmon, cod, scrod, haddock, halibut, flounder, sole, red snapper, brook trout, sea trout, and sea bass. Shellfish, such as lobster, shrimp, and clams, should be avoided, as should tunafish and swordfish.

Your other main meals of the week should be vegetarian. However, whole-wheat products should be eaten only once or twice a week, and grains should be limited to brown rice, barley, millet, and buckwheat. Good substitutes for grains are sweet or white baked potatoes, acorn or butternut squash, or Jerusalem artichokes.

Dairy products should be substantially reduced. *All* milks — raw, skim, or goats' — should be replaced by soy milk. Cottage, ricotta, or farmer's cheese should now be eaten only once or twice a week. Eggs should be reduced to two a week.

Fruits and vegetables now begin to play a prominent role in your diet. Fruit should be eaten two to three times a day between meals, or you may make an entire meals of fruits, eating, for instance, a whole cantaloupe or a large bowl of blueberries. Apples and apple juice, however, should now be eliminated, as should oranges, orange juice, pears, mangoes, and bananas. Such alkaline fruits as watermelon, papaya, grapefruit (an acidic fruit that has alkaline properties after digestion), honeydew, and cantaloupe are preferable choices for the A. Tomatoes, avocados, spinach, and cabbage should now be strictly eliminated from salads.

This diet should be followed for about three months.

Level Four

All meats should now be completely eliminated from your diet. However, if you have difficulty making this adjustment at this level, or if you are under physical stress and still require animal protein, eat fish two or three times a week. All lunches and dinners, barring these exceptions, should be vegetarian meals. All cheese and dairy products should now also be eliminated from your diet. Eggs should be reduced to one a week. Because the white of eggs is primarily albumin, which tends to create gas in the A, egg white should be cut away and only the yolk of the egg eaten.

All whole-wheat grains and wheat-derived products should now be eliminated. Only soy products should be eaten.

Pumpkin and sunflower seeds and almonds and brazil nuts should now become an integral part of your diet. Eat a handful of nuts or seeds a day as a source of protein. Sprouts from alfalfa, mung beans, lentils, and aduki seeds should become an important part of your diet because they are rich in minerals and also have a high vegetable protein content. Lima, soy, and kidney beans should be eaten for their protein. Eat a square of tofu four to five times a day.

Brown rice should be eaten only twice a week for it can be too acidic for the A.

Include a tablespoon of olive oil on your salads or steamed vegetables every day. It has a good nutrient value and aids in digestion and elimination.

This step should be worked into over a period of about four to five months.

Level Five

All meals should now be vegetarian. All grains and breads should be soy-derived. One egg may be eaten a week; all other dairy products should be eliminated from the diet. Brown rice may be eaten once or twice a week.

Seeds, sprouts, and tofu should be eaten every day as the main sources of protein. Fruits and vegetables are now the major source of all other nutrients.

This is the ideal menu for the A and the goal of your regimen. It should be worked into slowly, with great deliberation, and at your own pace.

Type B

Midway in characteristics between the A and O, the B has a tendency to react like an A with a catarrhal nature, or like an O in an unbalanced state of health. This condition I call Fatigued B. An inventory of your symptoms will reveal which way the regimen will be directed.

Level One

Regardless of your current physical tendencies, you should begin your program by eliminating processed and refined foods. Candies, soda pop, chocolate syrup, canned foods, and convenience dinners should be reduced as much as possible. Sugar should be replaced by honey. Whole grains should be substituted for instant and processed cereals. Introduce millet, soya/wheat, cornmeal, whole oats, or buckwheat into your diet. Whole-wheat products should be substituted for refined-flour products.

Beef and pork should be reduced as much as possible, substituting lamb, veal, chicken or turkey, and fish. Eggs should be organic and cheeses sould be made from raw goats' milk. Coffee and tea should be replaced by a coffee substitute such as Pero or Pioneer; and hard alcohol with red or white wine, preferably mixed half-and-half with charged water.

All fried and sautéed foods should now be eliminated. Meats and fish should always be eaten broiled or baked, eggs boiled or poached and vegetables steamed.

Your physical-exercise program should now also be examined. Your goal is a moderate program of activities such as jogging, swimming, hiking, bicycling, gymnastics, calisthenics, or Hatha Yoga. If your exercise program has been strenuous, reduce it now.

This level should be followed for about a month.

Level Two

Animal protein, such as veal, lamb, chicken, turkey, or fish, should be eaten once every day. Whole-wheat products should be alternated with soy products. Soy bread, soy wheat cereal, soy flakes and granules should be eaten four times a week, whole-wheat products, three. Tofu squares should be eaten four times a week.

Lunch should be vegetarian three times a week. Apple cider vinegar can be used with a polyunsaturated oil (safflower, sunflower, or soy) on salads twice a week; the other days lemon should be mixed in the dressing. Sea salt and kelp powder may be used in moderation as condiments.

Fruits should be eaten three times a day between meals. Alternate steamed and raw vegetables in order to allow the body to adapt to the laxative effect of raw vegetables.

You should now start reducing your dairy products. Soft cheeses such as ricotta, cottage, or farmer's cheese can be eaten four times a week, yogurt two or three times a week, and eggs should be cut back to five or six a week. If you use milk, drink raw cows' or goats' milk, but only four or five glasses a week. Start introducing soy milk as a milk substitute.

This diet should be followed for about two months.

Level Three

Depending upon whether the nature of your body is catarrhal (retaining a lot of mucus) or fatigued, you should follow one of these two diets.

Catarrhal Nature: Veal and lamb should be completely eliminated from your diet. Eat chicken or turkey once a week and fish twice a week. Recommended fish include: cod, flounder, red snapper, bluefish, halibut, salmon, sea trout, and sea bass. Shellfish should be avoided. Your other dinners should be vegetarian, for example, a salad, steamed vegetables, a sweet potato or a grain such as brown rice.

At this time do not eat whole-wheat products. Use soy products instead. Dairy foods should be greatly reduced and soy milk should replace raw cows' or goats' milk. You may eat soft cheeses only once or twice a week, and only two eggs a week. Tofu should be eaten four times a day.

Continue to eat fruit three times a day between meals. Apples and apple juice should be temporarily eliminated because of their high acidity level, and oranges, orange juice, bananas, and mangoes should also be avoided. Alkaline-forming fruits such as grapefruits, cantaloupe, and watermelon are better for you during this period. Lunches should be completely vegetarian.

Follow this diet for three to four months.

Fatigued B: Veal and lamb should be eaten once a week, chicken or turkey twice a week, and fish the remaining nights. Soft cheeses can be eaten three times a week, yogurt twice a week. You may have four to five eggs a week. A glass of cows' or goats' milk may be drunk three or four times a week.

You need to increase your protein intake, therefore, eat a square of tofu five times a day; and have soy protein drinks before breakfast and dinner (soy protein powder is available at any health food store). Stir a tablespoon-and-a-half of powder into a glass of water to make the drink.

Whole-wheat products may be alternated with soy products (whole wheat three times a week, soy, four times a week). Brown rice may be eaten two or three times a week, and other grains such as buckwheat, millet, or barley may also be eaten in place of brown rice. All lunches should now be vegetarian.

Olive oil should now be introduced into your diet to encourage proper digestion and healthy elimination. Take one tablespoon every other day.

Physical exercise should be reduced if your body is greatly fatigued; if not, an hour's exercise may be taken four times a week.

This regimen should be followed for three to four months, or until strength has been returned to your body.

Level Four

Catarrhal Nature: As the concentration of mucus is broken up and eliminated from your body, certain foods that were reduced or eliminated in level three may now be gradually re-introduced. Veal may again be eaten once a week. Chicken and turkey should now be eaten once or twice a week, and fish twice a week. The other main meals should be vegetarian.

Whole-wheat products, such as bread or soy/wheat cereal, may be eaten once a week. Grains such as millet, barley, or buckwheat should be re-introduced and eaten once a week. You may continue to eat brown rice once a week.

Soft cheeses may be eaten twice a week and yogurt once a week, and you may have three eggs a week. Two to three glasses of raw cows' or goats' milk per week may be re-introduced in your diet. Soy milk may be drunk as often as desired. You may now have apples and apple juice once a week. Oranges may also be eaten once a week. Lunches should be vegetarian.

Follow this diet for two to three months.

Fatigued B: As the fatigue abates and your body regains its strength you may have veal once a week and lamb once every two weeks. Chicken or turkey may be eaten once or twice a week, reduce your fish meals now to twice a week. All other dinners should be vegetarian.

You should now reduce your consumption of soft cheeses to twice a week, and yogurt to once a week. Whole milk should be diluted with water, and eventually be replaced by skim milk, skim milk diluted in water, and finally, soy milk. Four eggs may be eaten a week, and continue to eat tofu four or five times a day. The soy protein drinks can now be eliminated. However, if you experience brief periods of fatigue, re-introduce this supplement in your diet.

Stay on this diet for two months.

Level Five

At the ideal level, the B should eat chicken or turkey twice a week, fish twice a week, and vegetarian dinners three times a week. Every other week you may substitute calf's liver, lamb, or veal for fish or chicken. If your occupation is not demanding, the combination of vegetarian/meat meals can be meat or fish three nights and vegetarian four nights.

Soft cheeses may be eaten twice a week, and yogurt once a week. You may also eat three eggs a week and drink two or three glasses of whole milk a week.

Whole-wheat and soy products should be alternated: soy products four times a week, and whole-wheat products, three. You may have brown rice once or twice a week, and other grains such as millet, cornmeal, or barley once or twice weekly.

Apples and oranges can be eaten twice a week, but avoid bananas entirely.

Sea salt and kelp powder may be eaten as desired.

Type AB

Level One

At this initial level, you should begin by eliminating processed and refined foods and those with chemical preservatives, artificial flavorings, and additives. Coffee, tea, candies, soda pop, syrups, canned and prepared instant foods should now be reduced or eliminated. Bleached or enriched white-flour products should be replaced by whole-wheat products. Beef and pork products should be reduced, gradually being replaced by veal, lamb, chicken, turkey, and fish.

Eat only those dairy products made from raw cows' or goats' milk. Avoid commercially processed milk. Eggs should be fertile, and cold-pressed oil should be used instead of commercially refined oils.

Fried or sautéed foods should be eliminated. Meat and fish should be broiled or baked, vegetables steamed, and eggs soft-boiled or poached. Substitute red or white wine for hard alcohol, and reduce the amount of cigarettes you are smoking.

Evaluate your exercise program. Your goal, like the A, is a calming regimen. My recommended program includes Hatha Yoga, T'ai Chi Ch'uan, light jogging, hiking, swimming, or a gym workout.

Follow this diet for a month or two.

Level Two

Meats that may be eaten at this stage include veal, lamb, chicken, turkey, or fish. If possible your main meals should consist mostly of chicken or turkey and fish, instead of the more acidic meats, veal and lamb.

Whole-wheat products should now be alternated with soy products; whole wheat three and soy bread four times a week. Oatmeal, soy flakes, and soy granules are preferable to millet, farina, ground rice or corn. Wheat germ and bran should be limited to once or twice a week.

Eggs should be reduced to four a week. Whole milk should be diluted, eventually substituting first skim milk, then skim milk diluted with water, and, eventually, soy milk. Soft cheeses may be eaten two or three times a week, and yogurt twice a week.

Vegetables should be eaten steamed because if you are not accustomed to the laxative effect of raw vegetables your body needs time to adjust. Vegetarian meals should now be introduced at lunch (if this is not your main meal) at least two or three times a week.

Sea salt and kelp may be alternated as condiments. Apple cider vinegar should be eliminated. Use lemon juice instead with oil and herbs to dress vegetables or salads.

This diet should be followed for up to three months.

Level Three

Veal and lamb should now be completely eliminated from your diet. Eat chicken or turkey twice a week, and fish the other nights. Recommended fish include: cod, salmon, halibut, flounder, sole, red snapper, sea or brook trout, or sea bass. Shellfish and tuna and swordfish should be strictly avoided. If possible, introduce a vegetarian night once or twice a week and start cutting back slowly on your consumption of meat or fish.

Dairy products should now be slowly reduced. Raw milk should be replaced by soy milk. Soft cheeses should be reduced to twice a week, and yogurt to once a week. Eggs should be reduced to two a week.

Whole-wheat products should now be entirely eliminated. Substitute soy products. Grains such as millet, buckwheat, or barley should be reduced to once every two weeks. Brown rice may be eaten once or twice a week.

Fruits and vegetables should now begin to play a prominent part in your diet. Fruits should be eaten three or four times a day between meals. Apples and apple juice should be eliminated, as should oranges and orange juice, bananas, and mangoes. Vegetarian lunches should be increased to five or six a week, and vegetables may now be eaten both steamed and raw. An important addition to salads at this point are sprouted seeds including alfalfa, mung beans, lentils, and soy beans.

Take up to three months to work into this diet.

Level Four

Fish consumption should now be reduced to three times a week, and all other dinners should be vegetarian. All lunches should now also be vegetarian. Cheese and yogurt should be eliminated from your diet and butter replaced by soy, safflower, or lecithin margarine. All bread should be made from soy flour. Brown rice may be eaten once a week. Oatmeal and occasionally cornmeal may be eaten for breakfast.

Eat pumpkin and sunflower seeds and almonds every day for protein. Sprouts, which have a high mineral and protein content, should be an integral part of your daily diet. Mix them into salads or combine them with steamed vegetables. Lima, kidney, or soy beans should also be eaten for protein. One or two eggs may be eaten a week, but discard the white part, which is gas-forming to the AB.

Fruits and vegetables should comprise an ever-increasing part of your diet (in Europe it is not uncommon to have a plain salad for breakfast).

Follow this diet for about three months.

Level Five

The ideal AB is a vegetarian except for two meals a week that should include a variety of fish. All breads and grains should be soy derived, and dairy products must be strictly avoided. One or two eggs may be eaten a week. Eat seeds and almonds each day now. Sprouts, an important source of protein, should be eaten several times a day. You may have brown rice once a week, oatmeal every day, cornmeal twice a week, and bran once a week.

If you have a physically demanding occupation, you may want to add more fish or (occasionally) chicken to your diet to meet your energy requirements. This ideal level should be worked into at your own pace.

Although, as I have explained, different foods affect different blood types in dissimilar fashions, every nutrient possesses healing qualities. I have listed various foods that I recommend, with their healing qualities that I, as a practicing naturopath, have discovered. Some things, of course, are appropriate for certain blood types and not others. Check the diets in the last chapter.

7

VITAMINS AND
MINERALS

The word *vitamin* has only been in existence since 1911 when the Polish chemist Casimir Funk isolated the substance that later became known as Vitamin B_1. Funk called it the "beriberi vitamine." It has only been, then, in the last seventy-five years that people have recognized that vitamins are necessary for good health. Therefore, it should not be surprising that controversy still surrounds their use for healing. Orthodox physicians prefer drugs and surgery, despite the fact that these methods of healing are unnatural and intervene in the body's normal functioning.

Food, on the other hand, is a natural part of our lives. The fact that vitamins occur in food has quite possibly been one of the reasons orthodox medicine has ignored their healing properties. Orthodox physicians are more accustomed to healing with drugs and surgery than with tools derived from day-to-day life. This is not to say that scientists and medical people have not been looking into vitamins. Dr. Evan Shute and Dr. Linus Pauling are well known for their excellent research and their unwavering advocacy of vitamin therapy as a valid and effective healing technique. They belong to the growing camp of physicians who say that vitamins and minerals given in appropriate quantities can heal. So do I.

What's more, Recommended Dietary Allowances (RDA's) set by our governments require serious re-evaluation. Dietary needs of people today differ tremendously from those living sixty years ago when many of these standards were set. For example, our grandparents ate bread that contained 450 to 460 mg of Vitamin B complex. Not only does the white bread we eat today contain preservatives and gases, but it also contains not even one-tenth the amount of Vitamin B contained in our grandparents' bread. The amount of B complex that is there is synthetic.

I have been practicing natural healing methods for some thirty-five years now. In that time thousands of my patients have been helped. What made the difference in their conditions was the use of vitamin and mineral therapy. The diets I advocate will maintain excellent health in those who follow them. However, to get to the highest level of health possible, vitamin and mineral supplementation is nearly always necessary.

Most of us have not given our bodies adequate quantities of vitamins and minerals over the years. Tissues have therefore broken down, resulting in a varied array of illnesses. The food we eat is not concentrated enough to rebuild weaknesses in tissues and organs. Vitamin and mineral supplementation provides appropriate concentrations for rebuilding. Our food will only maintain appropriate concentrations for rebuilding. Our food will only maintain the body. Vitamins and minerals, if given in appropriate quantities, will repair weaknesses. As weaknesses are repaired, the need for additional vitamins and minerals decreases. However, people with stressful lives will always need supplementation as will those people who live in areas where there is little access to foods containing some vitamins and minerals. It is obvious, for example, that the requirements of the man who works on a construction site differ from those of the man who sits at a desk all day. Certainly, Olympic athletes are well aware of the importance of vitamin supplementation to their diets. In most countries of the world, trainers include extra vitamins and minerals in their athletes' training programs.

Let us look, for example, at an individual who has consumed three bottles of beer every day for ten years. This man is doing well in his work, has a comfortable income, a family of five, is a member of the local rotary club chapter, and coaches little league baseball.

He is not an alcoholic. He simply has a bottle of beer every day with his lunch as well as one before dinner and one later in the evening. If this man's diet does not contain adequate quantities of B vitamins, zinc, Vitamin C, magnesium, and amino acids, his health is at risk. All these vitamins and minerals have been found to be depleted following the ingestion of alcohol. Years of this daily drinking pattern will inevitably result in health problems if the individual has not taken adequate amounts of the above listed vitamins and minerals. Symptoms as seemingly unrelated as fatigue, constipation, kidney stones, atherosclerosis, and/or frequent colds may appear. Inevitably such symptoms will be explained away as being related to age or stress. In reality, this man has a vitamin and mineral deficiency. If the deficiency is not addressed, it is likely that far more serious symptoms will eventually develop. Such a result is never necessary. Proper diet can prevent this outcome. Vitamin and mineral supplementation can speed the reversal of it.

When I first assess patients, I usually advise large quantities of vitamin and mineral supplements. These amounts are often upsetting. However, within three to six months it is likely that the amount of supplementation will be reduced and, for some blood types, eliminated altogether within two years. At that time, simply eating proper foods will maintain excellent health. Only during the period of rebuilding weakened tissues do we need vitamin and mineral supplementation. They are, however, essential for reversal of health problems.

Vitamin A

This vitamin is primarily active in the cells that cover the outer and inner surfaces of the body. These include the skin and mucous membrances. As well, the lining of the mouth, the digestive tract, the urinary tract, and the respiratory tract are all affected by this vitamin. Adequate Vitamin A maintains them. Vitamin A is also essential for growth since it is necessary for proper formation of bones and the enamel on teeth. Because it is a component of the pigment that allows the eye to adjust to darkness after being exposed to bright light, it is closely associated with night vision. There is some research to suggest that Vitamin A is a stimulant to the immune system. Thus, it may very well be a powerful defense against viruses.

Vitamin-A deficiency is a worldwide problem. Mild deficiencies may show up in the form of acne or skin rashes. Dry, flaky skin as well as itchy eyes may mean that this essential vitamin is lacking. Loss of appetite or increased numbers of infections may also occur in a Vitamin-A deficient individual. Night blindness is, of course, a symptom of deficiency.

When the vitamin is lacking in large quantities, mucous membranes begin to dry up. In poverty-stricken nations thousands of children are blinded every year from Vitamin A shortages, for the mucous membranes of the eyes are among the first to dry up. Individuals who wear contact lenses often benefit from increased dosages of Vitamin A as it supports lubrication of the mucous membrane of the eye, making it easier to wear the lenses.

Because it lubricates the mucous membranes, it is useful in relieving joint pain. However, in order to affect such conditions, Vitamin A should be taken between meals. In combination with Vitamin C, this vitamin is useful in treatment of eye conditions, eczema, acne, impetago, boils, carbuncles, as well as lung and sinus conditions. It, along with vitamins C and E, is exceedingly beneficial to women who have uterus problems. It helps to repair the lining of the uterus as well as keep the tissue in this area healthy. Pregnant women need this vitamin, but the amount should be monitored by their physicians since an excessive dose can stain the liver.

Vitamin A is of equal value to all blood groups.

Since Vitamin A is a fat-soluble vitamin, cooking does not destroy the Vitamin A content of vegetables. The following foods are excellent sources of this vitamin: apricots, broccoli, cabbage, calf's liver, cantaloupe, carrots, celery, chard, cheese, cod liver oil, collards, dandelion greens, endive, fish, kale, lettuce, mustard greens, potatoes, squash, turnip greens, and watercress. In general, the deeper the color of the vegetable or fruit, the more Vitamin A is present.

Vitamin B

What was first viewed as Vitamin B is now known as the B-complex vitamins. These vitamins, which are essential in order for food to be transformed into energy, consist of thiamine, riboflavin, niacin, pyridoxine, cobalamin, pangamic acid, amygdalin, folic acid, pantothenic acid, biotin, choline, inosital, and PABA. Because B vitamins are involved in energy production, they are particularly important to the O blood types. O-types require more energy output than other types because they are primarily physical in nature. As the O-type increases physical activity, it is wise for him to make sure that he is eating foods rich in Vitamin B. Because Vitamin B is a water soluble vitamin, it is not stored in the body. Thus it is crucial that adequate amounts are received by the body each day. The B vitamins are more potent when taken together. They should be increased during times of stress.

These vitamins are found mainly in the outer husk of seeds and cereals and are completely lacking in bleached flour and polished rice. The following foods contain plentiful amounts of various B vitamins: almonds, asparagus, beans, brewer's yeast, buckwheat, cabbage, celery, corn, filberts, mustard greens, peanuts, rye germ, soy beans, spinach, tangerines, turnip greens, watercress, wheat germ, and whole-wheat products. Animal and dairy sources include cheese, eggs, liver, milk, and veal.

Thiamine (Vitamin B₁)

Thiamine is essential to proper functioning of the central nervous system. Milk deficiencies result in reduced stamina, depression, irritability, and inability to concentrate. Individuals who drink alcohol regularly or who eat large quantities of processed foods may find themselves depleted of thiamine and therefore exhibiting the above symptoms. Should the deficiency continue, fatigue, numbness in arms or legs, cramps, and even weight loss can set in. In North America, we rarely see extreme forms of thiamine deficiency because small quantities are available in various foods. Instead, people develop small degrees of deficiency symptomology. They may show stiffness, tingling, and some numbness from time to time. Because such symptoms are non-specific, they are usually ignored. They do, however, significantly reduce the quality of life available to many people.

In the nineteenth century, when Western traders brought polished rice to the Orient, beriberi set in. The people had replaced their whole-grain brown rice with the white rice that had the thiamine-rich hull removed. Beriberi is characterized by a progression from stiffness in the legs, through numbness and tingling, to paralysis, and ultimately muscle atrophy.

Thiamine aids in the digestion of carbohydrates. It is also helpful in the treatment of herpes zoster as well as being a useful tool for combating air sickness.

Type O requires a higher level of thiamine; Type B a lower level, and Type A a miniscule amount.

Foods rich in thiamine include brown rice, eggs, green leafy vegetables, liver, peanuts, wheat germ, whole grain cereals, and yeast.

Riboflavin (Vitamin B₂)

Riboflavin is necessary for energy release. It is also used to promote growth and tissue repair, and it supports healthy nails, hair, and skin. It should be increased during pregnancy and lactation. Although there has not been as yet a great deal of research into minor deficiencies of this vitamin, some studies suggest a relationship to rheumatoid arthritis, depression, and cataracts. Frequently I see a minor deficiency of riboflavin in people who have either hypoglycemia or a sugar intolerance. Symptoms of severe deficiency include cracking and inflammation at the edges of the lips, a purple tongue, swollen membranes in the mouth and throat as well as irritable, tearing, bloodshot eyes. A rash can appear on the face and growth in children may be interrupted.

Like thiamine, riboflavin is required more by Type O, less by Type B, and hardly at all by Type A.

Milk is high in riboflavin and used to be our usual source of the vitamin. However, the pasteurization process destroys the B-complexes as well as the Vitamin C that occurs in it naturally. Moreover, since riboflavin is destroyed in light, milk and milk products should not be stored in clear containers unless they are kept in the dark. After two hours of exposure to direct sunlight, milk can lose 50 to 70 percent of its riboflavin. Other foods high in riboflavin include broccoli, collard greens, eggs, fish, green vegetables, kidney, liver, mushrooms, and okra.

Niacin (Vitamin B₃)

Nicotinic acid, niacinamide, niacin, or Vitamin B_3 is the vitamin that began the raging controversy surrounding mega-vitamin therapy in 1952. Niacin had by that time been acknowledged as essential in the prevention of pellagra, a disease common in the poverty-stricken southern American states during the early part of the twentieth century. Skin, digestive tract, and tissues of the nervous system are affected by a deficiency of this vitamin. Thus, severe skin rashes, diarrhea, psychosis, and eventually death can result.

Then two Canadian psychiatrists, Drs. Abram Hoffer and Humphrey Osmond, became fascinated by the dementia that accompanies severe niacin deficiency and wondered if it could be connected to schizophrenia and other mental illnesses. Using large doses of the substance, they received remarkable results with thousands of patients. The anti-vitamin camp of physicians, does not, of course, accept their results. However, a growing number of physicians do acknowledge their pioneering in the field.

In one very interesting study, Dr. Hoffer examined 1,150 people who had been accused of some criminal act. Of people who had pellagra, 27 percent were accused of murder. Of those who did not have the deficiency, only 10 percent were accused of the crime. Another finding of his study was that more than one-third of all murderers diagnosed as insane had pellagra. There is, then, some possibility that violent crime could be reduced by simply screening people for niacin deficiency.

Minor deficiencies of niacin show up as irritability, headaches, dizziness, inner-ear problems, insomnia, occasional diarrhea, and other digestive disturbances. Recently, large doses have been used in the treatment of hyperactivity in children as well as of learning disorders. Dependency on nicotine, alcohol, and drugs have been helped by mega-doses of niacin. There is even some evidence that arthritis can be helped by this vitamin.

This vitamin dilates, or opens up, the blood vessels. When first taken as a supplement, it may cause itchiness and what appears to be a heat rash. This is really the drug taking effect. Small blood vessels are opening up. Minor deficiencies constrict blood vessels and poor circulation to the brain results in a lack of mental alertness or depression. Small problems become big ones because it takes more mental effort to solve them. Correcting the deficiency will increase mental clarity, and the depression will ease up. The vitamin is also helpful in maintaining good skin and a healthy digestive tract. It affects the pancreas and adrenals, will assist in lowering high blood pressure, and will increase energy.

The amount needed of this vitamin depends on a person's condition and symptoms, not blood type.

Foods abundant in niacin include cottage cheese, dates, figs, kidney, lean meats, legumes, liver, soybeans, tofu, and wheat germ.

Pyridoxine (Vitamin B_6)

Pyridoxine is essential in protein metabolism and is necessary for the production of red blood cells and the proper functioning of nervous system tissue. Many North Americans may be deficient in this vitamin as it is destroyed by heating. Furthermore, the milling process used to make white flour and processed foods removes Vitamin B_6. It appears to be a natural diuretic and can be useful when given in high doses for individuals who retain water. It is also very good for pregnant women who have morning sickness. Mega-vitamin doses have been given to correct conditions as widely varied as acne and ulcers. It is also useful to promote growth and appetite in young children. Because it is an oxidant, B_6 is used to promote circulation. In combination with other vitamins, it is useful in reducing the numbers of atherosclerotic plaques and cholesterol buildup. Women who take the birth control pill should increase intake of Vitamin B_6.

Nervous disorders as well as anemia result from a B_6 deficiency. Skin rashes and sore mouth and tongue can also result. Serious deficiencies may cause a wide variety of symptoms: these include nausea, vomiting, weight loss, mental confusion, anemia, kidney stones, and even convulsions in children. Alcohol consumption is a contributing factor to Vitamin B_6 deficiencies. There is as yet no known reason for this phenomenon, but heavy drinkers are wise to include Vitamin B_6 supplements in their diets.

All blood types require this vitamin.

Foods high in Vitamin B_6 include bananas, blackstrap molasses, brewer's yeast, cantaloupe, eggs, kale, legumes, liver, rice bran, soybeans, spinach, and wheat germ.

Cobalamin (Vitamin B_{12})

Vitamin B_{12} is essential for proper production of cells since it is necessary for the synthesis of DNA and RNA. Thus, almost any area in the body is likely to be affected by severe deficiency. However, the most commonly affected parts are the digestive tract, the production of red blood cells, and the nervous system. Conditions such as fatigue and lowered resistance can therefore be alleviated by this vitamin. It may also be of benefit prior to and during menstruation.

Mild deficiencies may result in digestive upsets and constipation or diarrhea. More severe deficiencies cause pernicious anemia and central nervous system deterioration, including paralysis, psychosis, and ultimately death.

Because cobalamin is stored well in the body, deficiencies may not show up for three or four years. Vegetarians are most at risk because most sources of the vitamin are found in animal products. Therefore, those following a Type-A diet need more than others.

Lean meats and dairy products are the best natural sources for this vitamin. To be most effective, B_{12} should be combined with calcium and folic acid.

Pangamic Acid (Vitamin B_{15})

The vitamin is rarely used as a supplement in North America, although it is widely prescribed in Russia. It has been found to be helpful in heart disease, alcoholism, and diabetes. Since it is an anti-oxidant (it keeps oxygen in the bloodstream), it is used by athletes. Deficiency will result in glandular and nerve disorders.

Vitamin B_{15} is found in brown rice, whole grains, pumpkin seeds, and sesame seeds.

Laetrile (Vitamin B_{17} or Amygdalin)

This vitamin is at present the center of tremendous controversy in the fight to find a cure for cancer. German and Mexican researchers have documented many successes in treating cancer victims if the vitamin is used in combination with other forms of chemotherapy; but there is minimal acceptance of this cure in North America. There is, however, some acceptance of its effectiveness in the treatment of sickle-cell anemia. This vitamin is extracted from the seeds of many fruits, in particular, the apricot seed. Pits of cherries, nectarines, peaches, and plums, also contain this vitamin.

Folic Acid

Like Vitamin B_{12}, folic acid is important for the formation of DNA and RNA. Because folic acid is easily destroyed by cooking or canning, there is a widespread mild deficiency in North Americans who are fond of processed foods. Alcoholics are usually deficient in folic acid as they cannot absorb it. Pregnant women need to be particularly careful to have enough of it in their diets as it is necessary for the growth of the fetus. Folic acid can protect against parasites and food poisoning and therefore is a useful vitamin to take when traveling. As well as anemia, mild to moderate deficiencies cause irritability, forgetfulness, weakness, tiredness, diarrhea, headache, and even palpatations. Severe deficiencies can result in depression and psychosis.

Uncooked or lightly cooked fruits or vegetables provide an ample supply of this vitamin. Legumes are rich in folic acid, as are green leafy vegetables like spinach and romaine lettuce. Beets, broccoli, brussels sprouts, and cabbage all contain large amounts of the vitamin. Cantaloupe and oranges contain folic acid, as do yeast and brewer's yeast. Other sources are egg yolks, dark rye flour, and liver.

Pantothenic Acid

This vitamin is key to energy metabolism and is found in every living cell. Since it is also present in high quantities in adrenal gland tissues, it may be helpful in conditions where steroids might otherwise be used, including such illnesses as allergies, asthma, and arthritis. Because of this association with the adrenal glands, pantothenic acid is instrumental in promoting the production of antibodies used to fight infections.

This vitamin may be especially useful to relax neck and shoulder muscles, which tend to be tense in Type A's.

Pantothenic acid is destroyed by freezing and by processing techniques. It is found in ample quantities in whole grains and legumes. Broccoli, lentils, molasses, and soybeans are also high in the vitamin.

Biotin

This vitamin works in connection with enzymes in the many processes that produce energy. It works with vitamins A, B_2, B_6, and niacin in maintaining healthy skin. Deficiencies are rare, as biotin is made by intestinal bacteria. The only threat would be raw eggs eaten in a quantity of ten a day (the egg white prevents absorption of biotin). Those who drink lots of egg nog need to be aware of this possible deficiency.

Fruits, nuts, and brewer's yeast are other sources of biotin.

Choline

Choline is a fat emulsifier that, in conjunction with inositol, is essential for the utilization of fats and cholesterol. It helps control cholesterol build-up and promotes memory, especially in later years. There is some thought that a deficiency of this vitamin may be a contributing factor in Alzheimer's disease.

Choline is found in egg yolk, green leafy vegetables, liver, and wheat germ.

Inositol

Inositol is important in muscle cell growth and may well be a preventive vitamin for the development of atherosclerotic plaques. There is some indication, too, that it reduces baldness as well as preventing eczema. High dosages have been found to be a mild tranquilizer as well as an effective sedative. It is one of the constituents lost in the refining of flour, and thus whole-wheat products are good sources of this vitamin. Other sources include cabbage, cantaloupe, grapefruit, organ meats, and raisins.

PABA

PABA helps in the formation of folic acid and is important in the utilization of protein. Large doses combat fatigue. It is a membrane stabilizer and seems to have the ability to protect against ozone toxicity. It may therefore be beneficial to people who live in smoggy areas. It is also an effective sunscreen, now widely used in suntan oils. There is some indication that it reduces hair loss. It keeps skin healthy and smooth, and delays the formation of wrinkles.

This vitamin is found in brewer's yeast, lean meats, molasses, and whole grains.

Vitamin C
(Ascorbic Acid)

Vitamin C is by far the most talked about vitamin. It is recognized by most people as being the anti-cold vitamin. It is an essential ingredient of collagen, the connective tissue that literally sticks our body together. Thus bones and teeth need large quantities of Vitamin C for repairs, and wound healing is enhanced by extra quantities. When tissues have low quantities of Vitamin C in them they are more vulnerable to infections. Thus it has been demonstrated repeatedly that, in large doses, Vitamin C can contribute to reducing the frequency and the severity of colds. This point is still, however, a bone of contention for many oxthodox physicians.

Other beneficial effects of the vitamin include immune system stimulus as well as protection against atherosclerosis. There is also some evidence that Vitamin C helps protect the body against carcinogens, such as nitrites, thus reducing the risk of cancer. Smokers are advised to take supplements of Vitamin C, as each cigarette smoked depletes the body of 25 mg of this valuable protective vitamin. Vitamin C is also a useful substance to take in order to reduce stress reactions. It is frequently used to promote healing following surgery. It is a natural laxative and may assist in preventing clotting of veins.

We are all, of course, aware of ascorbic acid's use in the prevention of scurvy. A mild Vitamin C deficiency can produce some bleeding of the gums, reduced endurance, listlessness, and occasional joint pain. Moderate deficiency causes easy bruising of the skin and rupturing of small blood vessels. Asthma, sinus, and respiratory conditions are often related to Vitamin C deficiencies.

Vitamin C is not stored in the body nor is it manufactured by the body as it is by animals. We must, then, always be sure to take enough. However, it is unstable. Vitamin C is water soluble and is destroyed by heat, and even by the metals in iron and copper pans. Thirty seconds after an orange is picked from the tree, approximately 87 percent of its Vitamin C content is lost. Milk, which at one time was a whole food containing large quantities of Vitamin C, no longer carries that vitamin in it because it is destroyed in the process of pasteurization.

Type O's require large amount of Vitamin C than do Type A's (who require a modified amount) and B (who require even less). Specific ailments also call for larger dosages at the discretion of the physician.

Food sources for Vitamin C include broccoli, brussels sprouts, cantaloupe, cauliflower, collard greens, grapefruit, green pepper, guava, kale, oranges, papaya, potatoes, red pepper, sorrel, and sweet potatoes.

Vitamin D

We are familiar with the "sunshine vitamin." Sunshine alters a substance in our skin into a substance that the kidney can change into Vitamin D. This vitamin is essential for strong and rigid bones. It monitors the use of calcium and phosphorus. If there is a deficiency of Vitamin D, calcium and phosphorus cannot be used by the bones even if there is an excess of these minerals. The result of deficiency is tooth decay, bone diseases, and, ultimately, rickets. Because Vitamin D is stored in the liver, adult requirements are usually met. However, smog does affect the amount of sunshine that reaches cities, and thus city-dwellers ought to take extra Vitamin D. In children, Vitamin D is crucial to growth.

High doses of this vitamin can produce toxicity. A safe dose is 400 to 1000 I.U.'s. At present, most milk and milk products are fortified with Vitamin D. This amount seems to look after requirements for most North Americans. Vitamin D is stable and survives cooking, processing, and storing. Good sources of Vitamin D are fish oils, herring, salmon, sardines, and tuna.

Vitamin E

The controversy surrounding the therapeutic value of Vitamin E has been raging since 1935 when Dr. Evan Shute of London, Ontario, first discovered the value of this vitamin in the treatment of hemorrhage following abortion. Dr. Shute tirelessly investigated Vitamin E throughout his life, using strict and valid scientific techniques. Nevertheless, his findings have been largely ignored by the orthodox medical community. However, considerable scientific documentation has been building up from all over the world, and some time in the next fifty years this valuable substance will have to be acknowledged for its ability to treat and prevent many heart conditions (including angina) as well as its amazing ability to heal burns without scarring, to treat varicose veins, and to care for individuals suffering from diabetes. It is also used to reduce blood cholesteral levels. Women benefit from this vitamin throughout pregnancy, lactation, and menopause. Those who take birth control pills should also take Vitamin E.

Vitamin E is an anti-oxidant, preventing the oxidation of fat compounds and protecting cell membranes from breaking down and, therefore, keeping them strong. It enhances the action of Vitamin A and is a vasodilator and anti-coagulant. Individuals with high blood pressure should not take Vitamin E for this reason.

Vitamin E occurs naturally in vegetable oils and in whole grains. Unfortunately, it is one of the nutrients removed from wheat during refining and, consequently, is not contained in white bread for, unlike the B vitamins, which are also removed, it is not replaced. Since bread used to be a main source of Vitamin E, the loss has surely affected the health of North Americans over the last seventy years.

Deficiency levels are not clear since those who established the levels based them on the amounts of the vitamin that average Americans carry in their bodies. Unfortunately, these "average" Americans were those who ate refined breads and oils, which had had much of the vitamin content removed.

Cold pressed vegetable oils and whole grains are our best sources of Vitamin E. Wheat germ and wheat-germ oil contain very high quantities of Vitamin E.

Vitamin K

Since Vitamin K is necessary for the clotting of blood, it can assist in reducing excessive menstrual flow, and it may be a preventive against internal bleeding or hemorrhages. Deficiency results in celiac disease. It is synthesized by bacteria in the intestine. Food sources include alfalfa dark-green leafy vegetables, egg yolk, liver, soybean oil, and yogurt.

Calcium

In conjunction with phosphorus, calcium is necessary for the building of bones and teeth. It is essential in the normal clotting of blood and for proper growth. It promotes normal responses of muscles and nerves and is beneficial in relieving stress and depression. Calcium also supports proper sleeping habits since it calms and relaxes the body. In combination with magnesium, it promotes cardiovascular health. Low calcium intake can result in osteoporosis, the brittle bones of old age. Interestingly, it is thought that this condition may be, in part, a result of too much protein in the diet. However, I do not agree with this point of view.

There are many forms of calcium including bonemeal, calcium acetate, calcium gluconate, calcium lactate, chelated calcium, and dolomite. Some blood types absorb some forms of calcium better than others. Type A's, for example, absorb calcium lactate and calcium gluconate best, while Type O's can usually manage any form. Women, especially those in menopause, require more calcium than men.

Sources of calcium include asparagus, almonds, beans, beets, cabbage, carrots, cauliflower, celery, dairy products, greens, kale, soybeans, and sunflower seeds.

Chlorine

Chlorine regulates the blood's acid-alkaline level. There is rarely a deficiency in our diets as it is found in table salt. Other sources include olives and kelp. Chlorine can lower blood pressure and seems to be a deterrent for diabetes.

Chromium

Chromium stimulates enzymes in the production of energy. It further assists in the synthesis of protein, cholesterol, and fatty acids. It is thought to increase the effectiveness of insulin.

Deficiencies slow down the group rate as well as contribute to sugar intolerance and high blood cholesterol. Food sources include brewer's yeast, clams, corn oil, meats, and shellfish. It is helpful to know whether or not the soil from which your vegetables come is low in chromium. If this is the case, chromium supplements should be part of the diet.

Cobalt

Cobalt is a constituent of Vitamin B_{12}. It is essential in the prevention of anemia and rheumatic diseases.

Foods that contain cobalt include fish, leafy vegetables, legumes, liver, and whole cereals.

Copper

Copper is necessary for many enzyme reactions. It helps in the formation of hemoglobin and is useful in the treatment of arthritis. Only minute quantities of this mineral are needed. Excesses can result in insomnia, depression, and headaches. There may also be some relationship with schizophrenia. Increased levels of zinc will often counteract such symptoms.

Copper is found in bran, fish, leafy vegetables, liver, mushrooms, nuts, peas, poultry, and whole grains.

Iodine

This mineral promotes health of the thyroid gland. It provides an essential ingredient for the thyroid hormone. Indeed, two-thirds of the body's iodine content is found in the thyroid gland. It is essential for metabolism. Iodine deficiency can cause goiter.

Sources of iodine include bran, broccoli, butter, carrots, cherries, corn, fish, kelp, oats, onions, sea plants, and spinach.

Iron

Iron is essential to the enzyme systems that carry oxygen. It is thus very important to the body as the cells burn oxygen in order to produce energy. This valuable mineral, which is found in high concentrations in hemoglobin, is essential in the development of red blood cells. It is also found in muscle tissue, which, of course, has a high energy output. It aids in growth, is useful in promoting resistance to disease, and promotes good skin tone.

As food refinement increased in this century and people gave up cooking in cast iron pots (which added iron to the food cooked in them), more and more people became deficient in iron. Iron deficiency is now common all over the world, including North America. Symptoms include, weakness, pale skin, reduced appetite, mild depression, dizziness, and chronic fatigue.

Foods that contain large quantities of iron include almonds, asparagus, beans, celery, chard, cauliflower, currants, dandelion, egg yolk, fish, hearts, kale, kidney, liver, and prune juice.

Lysine

Lysine is one of the amino acids. These substances form protein compounds and are found in flesh foods. As well, and in varying degrees, they are found in products from the vegetable kingdom. All too often people forget this. Nature has provided us with a perfect solution. Type A's lean toward the vegetable kingdom. Many physicians believe that the vegetarian has trouble receiving amino acids and Vitamin B_{12}. Thus they view vegetarianism as dangerous. My view is that the danger exists only for a Type-O individual who is trying to be a vegetarian. The amino acid compounds found in vegetables are not strong enough to support a Type-O person. Flesh foods are required. The Type-A person, on the other hand, has a very different body than the Type O. Type-A harmonics are much lower than Type O's. Amino acids found in flesh foods are overabundant for the Type A. Legumes, nuts, seeds, and soya products can provide a Type A with ample amino acids. Vegetarianism will not deplete the body of the Type A.

Magnesium

Magnesium is an activator for many enzyme systems. It is necessary for proper metabolism of calcium and phosphorus, Vitamin C, sodium, and potassium. Considerable amounts of this mineral are deposited in bones, and it is required for the contraction of muscles as well as for conduction of impulses throughout the nervous system. It is an anti-stress vitamin and necessary for a healthy cardiovascular system.

Deficiencies commonly occur among heavy drinkers. High sugar intake has been implicated as well. Long-term diuretic therapy can also result in a deficiency. Refinement of bread and softening of water are further contributors to magnesium loss in our diets. Minor deficiencies can result in irritability, dizziness, high blood pressure, muscle weakness, and heart problems.

Good sources of magnesium include almonds, barley, beans, beet greens, brazil nuts, brown rice, carrots, cashews, chard, corn, dandelion, figs, fish, grapefruit, hazel nuts, lemons, oatmeal, peas, potatoes, walnuts, whole wheat, and watercress.

Manganese

Manganese promotes growth and is necessary for a healthy reproductive system as well as the central nervous system. It also works closely with enzymes and is a factor in thyroid function. It is necessary for proper digestion and for proper use of Vitamin B_1 and Vitamin C. Manganese improves memory and reduces irritability.

Food sources include almonds, beans, beets, bran, chard, eggs, peas, leafy greens, and whole grains.

Nickel

Nickel helps the body digest sugar. It can be found in bean sprouts, celery, garlic, lettuce, onions, seaweed, and string beans.

Phosphorus

Phosporus works in combination with calcium and Vitamin D to build strong bones. Phosphorus helps maintain alkalinity in the blood and is necessary for the digestion of carbohydrates and fats. Because Type A's lack hydrochloric acid, I do not suggest that they take calcium with phosphorus in it as this would lower their acid levels even more. Phosphorus is necessary for good kidney and nervous system functioning. It will give you energy and vitality and may be helpful in reducing the pain of arthritis. Deficiencies result in soft or brittle bones. Too much of this mineral, on the other hand, can throw off mineral balance and especially cause decreased calcium levels.

Phosphorus is found in almonds, barley, beans, bran, cheese, eggs, corn, fish, lentils, liver, milk, peas, poultry, and whole wheat.

Potassium

Potassium is an essential ingredient of the blood, the brain, and the nerve cells. Deficiencies can occur following prolonged vomiting and diarrhea, sunstroke, burns, hypoglycemia, diuretic therapy, and prolonged fasting. Weakness and mental confusion may result. This is one of the minerals responsible for maintaining proper fluid balance in the body. Potassium can assist in reducing high blood pressure and may be helpful in the treatment of some allergies.

Individuals with Type A need more minerals, especially potassium, in the summer when they tend to become dehydrated, which throws their electrolytes off.

Good sources of potassium include bananas, beans, beets, bran, cabbage, celery, lettuce, parsnips, potatoes, spinach, and sunflower seeds.

Selenium

Selenium is one of the trace minerals. It has been found to be an immune system stimulant. It works in combination with Vitamin E in such a way that the two substances potentiate each other. It is an anti-oxidant and may have properties that reduce hair loss and dandruff. It is also thought to prevent the aging of tissues. Males seem to need more selenium than females as almost 50 percent of the body's supply is found in the testicles. There is some thought that this mineral may alleviate some of the more distressing symptoms of menopause, such as hot flushes. Large quantities of this mineral may be toxic.

Food sources include wheat, whole grains, bran, onions, tomatoes, and broccoli. As with chromium, the soil in some areas of the country is selenium deficient. If possible, find out if this is the case for areas growing the vegetables you eat. It may be necessary to take selenium supplements if the soil is depleted of this vital mineral.

Sulphur

Sulphur occurs in some of the amino acids. It is necessary for the proper functioning of nerves and helps in the building of cells. It tones skin and fights infection. Sulphur is necessary for healthy hair, skin, and nails.

Beans, cabbage, chard, cheese, eggs, fish, lean meats, peas, oats, onions, and watercress, are good sources of sulphur.

Sodium

Sodium is necessary for the maintenance of body fluid balance. It maintains osmotic pressure — the balance of pressure in blood vessels, lymph glands, and tissues. Excessive sodium intake over a long period of time can result in hypertension and eventually in strokes. Addition of salt to foods is not necessary. North Americans who use a great deal of table salt as well as that already added to processed foods risk upsetting the fluid balance of their bodies. Because the concentrations of sodium become too high in the bloodstream, the kidneys retain water rather than excrete it in order to maintain a proper concentration of sodium. This large amount of fluid in the bloodstream creates a tension between small blood vessels, which constrict to keep the cells from holding too much water, and the large arteries and veins, which are then overloaded. Such stress to the cardiovascular system creates many health problems.

Read labels on packaged foods. The words *sodium, soda, salt,* or the symbol *Na* means that sodium has been added to the food. These are not necessary additives from a nutritional standpoint and, indeed, can be considered dangerous. We are best to avoid adding salt to food. Adequate amounts occur naturally in much of what we eat. Beets, carrots, celery, chard, cheese, eggs, olives, spinach, turnip, watercress, and wheat germ all contain large quantities of sodium.

Silicon

Silicon is necessary for the proper growth of hair, nails, and teeth. It is found in asparagus, beets, carrots, cherries, endive, figs, fruits with skin, peas, tomatoes, watermelon, and whole wheat.

Tryptophan

This amino acid is widely used as a sedative by those who wish to avoid the use of narcotic sedatives. It also stimulates growth-hormone release and assists in memory retention.

Zinc

Zinc is essential for the growth and repair of tissues. It sparks vitamin activity, aids tissue respiration, and corrects insulin function. It maintains the acid/alkaline balance and may reduce cholesterol buildup. Zinc affects brain function and is sometimes used in the treatment of schizophrenia. It is useful in correcting prostate conditions.

Because much zinc is removed in milling, refining, and canning, deficiencies are not uncommon. In children, a zinc deficiency can result in loss of appetite, failure to grow, and immaturely developed sexual organs. Lack of zinc slows wound healing. People who drink large quantities of alcohol deplete zinc reserves as it is necessary for the detoxification process. While spots on fingernails may indicate low zinc levels.

Food sources of zinc include broccoli, brown rice, dandelion, eggs, ground mustard, herring, legumes, lentils, liver, peas, pumpkin seeds, spinach, watercress, wheat, wheat bran, wheat germ, and yeast.

8

VITAMINS AND MINERALS FOR BLOOD TYPES

The following recommendations are for those who are maintaining a proper diet and are under minimal stress. Changes to these amounts may be made under certain conditions. Increased B-complex vitamins are needed by an individual under unusual stress. Vitamin C can be increased if an individual feels a cold coming or is under unusual stress. Because physical conditions vary so dramatically between individuals, a more personalized vitamin program aimed at an individual's specific strengths and weaknesses can really be determined only by a physician familiar with vitamin and mineral therapy. I highly recommend seeing such a person for advice if you wish to heal yourself in a natural way.

Type O

Vitamin A: 10,000 I.U. once a day
Vitamin B: one high potency stress B-complex tablet per day:
$\quad\quad$ 100 mg of B_1
$\quad\quad$ 100 mg of B_2

100 mg of B_6
20 mg of B_3
500 mcg of B_{12}

Pantothenic acid: 250 mg once to twice daily when under stress
Folic acid: 800 mcg daily
Vitamin C: 1000 mg once to twice daily (more if needed)
Vitamin D: 400 mg daily
Vitamin E: 400 I.U. daily
Iron: one tablet daily (use homeopathic iron if this causes
    constipation)
Bonemeal, chelated calcium, or calcium gluconate: 500 to 1000
    mg per day (women generally need 1000 mg or more)
Multi-mineral tablet: 1 to 2 daily

Type A

Vitamin A: 10,000 I.U. daily
Vitamin B: one or two low stress B-complex tablets daily (not
made from yeast, made from rice polishing powder)

(**N.B.** High stress B-complex pills could cause toxicity in Type A's.)
5 to 10 mg of B_1
5 to 10 mg of B_2
10 mg of B_3
100 to 500 mcg of B_{12}
50 mg of B_6

Folic acid: 400 mcg daily
Vitamin C: 250 mg daily (More may be taken if a cold occurs,
    but on relief of symproms, dosage should be reduced
    as continued excessive use can cause problems in
    the body.)
Vitamin D: 400 mg daily
Vitamin E: 200 I.U. daily
Glutamic acid hydrochloric: 1 to 2 tablets once a day (or 1/4 rennet
                                    tablet)

Calcium lactate or Calcium gluconate: 500 mg daily for men;
1000 mg for women

Multi-mineral tablet: 1 to 2 daily

Digestive enzyme: one tablet daily with the heaviest meal

Kelp tablets: 2 to 3 daily

Type B

Vitamin A: 10,000 I.U. daily

Vitamin B: 1 to 2 B-complex vitamin tablets daily:

         100 mg of B_1

         100 mg of B_2

          10 mg of B_3

          50 mg of B_6

         1 to 2 100 mg tablets of B_{12} every day

Folic acid: 400 mcg daily

Vitamin C: 250 mg twice a day

Vitamin D: 400 mg daily

Vitamin E: 400 I.U. daily

Multi-mineral tablet: 1 to 2 daily

Calcium gluconate or Bonemeal: 2 to 3 tablets daily (about
1000 mg)

Iron: one tablet every three days

Type AB

Vitamin A: 10,000 I.U. daily

Vitamin B: 1 to 2 low potency B-complex tablet every day:

          5 to 10 mg of B_1

          5 to 10 mg of B_2

         10 mg of B_3

         50 mg of B_6

         100 to 500 mcg of B_{12}

Folic acid: 400 mcg daily

Vitamin C: 250 mg daily

Vitamin D: 400 mg daily
Vitamin E: 200 mg twice a day
Calcium gluconate or Calcium lactate: 500 mg daily
Kelp: two tablets every day
Multi-mineral tablet: 1 to 2 daily
Glutamic acid hydrochloric: one tablet daily (or 1/4 rennet tablet)
Iron: every 10 days
Enzyme: one tablet following a heavy meal

Type Oa

Vitamin A: 10,000 I.U. daily
Vitamin B: one high potency stress B-complex daily:

$\quad\quad$ 100 mg of B_1
$\quad\quad$ 100 mg of B_2
$\quad\quad\ \ $ 20 mg of B_3
$\quad\quad$ 100 mg of B_6
$\quad\quad$ 500 mg of B_{12}

Folic acid: 800 mcg daily
Pantothenic acid: 250 mg daily
Vitamin C: 1500 mg daily (more if needed)
Vitamin D: 400 mg daily
Vitamin E: 400 I.U. daily
Iron: one tablet daily (use homeopathic iron if this causes
$\quad$ constipation)
Calcium gluconate: 500 to 1000 mg daily (women should take at
least 1000 mg a day)
Multi-mineral tablet: 1 to 2 daily

Type Ob

Vitamin A: 10,000 I.U. daily
Vitamin B: one high potency stress B-complex daily:

100 mg of B_1
100 mg of B_2
20 mg of B_3
100 mg of B_6
500 mcg of B_{12}

Folic acid: 800 mcg daily
Pantothenic acid: 250 mg 1 to 2 daily when under stress
Vitamin C: 1000 mg 1 to 2 daily (more if needed)
Vitamin D: 400 mg daily
Vitamin E: 400 I.U. every day
Iron: one tablet daily (use homeopathic iron if this causes
   constipation)
Bonemeal, Chelated calcium, or Calcium gluconate: 500 to
   1000 mg daily (women require at least 1000 mg)
Multi-mineral tablet: 1 to 2 daily

Type Ao

Vitamin A: 10,000 I.U. daily
Vitamin B: 1½ High stress B tablets every day (1 tablet in morning
1/2 tablet in the evening):
100 mg of B_1
100 mg of B_2
20 mg of B_3
100 mg of B_6
500 mcg of B_{12}

Folic acid: 400 mcg daily
Vitamin C: 1000 mg daily
Vitamin D: 400 mg daily
Vitamin E: 400 I.U. daily
Glutamic acid hydrochloric: 1 to 2 tablets once a day (or 1/4 of a
                              rennet tablet once a day)
Calcium lactate or Calcium glutamate: 500 mg daily for men;
                              1000 mg for women
Multi-mineral tablet: 1 to 2 daily
Digestive enzyme: one tablet daily with the heaviest meal
Kelp tablets: one daily

Type Ab

Vitamin A: 10,000 I.U. daily
Vitamin B: 3 low stress B-complex tablets every day:
        5 to 10 mg of B_1
        5 to 10 mg of B_2
        10 mg of B_3
        50 mg of B_6
        100 to 500 mcg of B_{12}
Folic acid: 400 mcg daily
Vitamin C: 500 to 700 mg daily
Vitamin D: 400 mg daily (Canada)
        800 mg daily (U.S.A.)
Vitamin E: 200 I.U. daily
Glutamic acid hydrochloric: 1 to 2 tablets once a day (or 1/4 of a
        rennet tablet)
Calcium lactate or Calcium gluconate: 500 to 700 mg daily
Multi-mineral tablet: 1 to 2 every day
Digestive enzyme: one tablet daily with the heaviest meal
Kelp tablets: 2 to 3 daily

Type Bo

Vitamin A: 10,000 I.U. daily
Vitamin B: Two high stress B-complex tablets every day:
        100 mg of B_1
        100 mg of B_2
        20 mg of B_3
        50 mg of B_6
        100 to 200 mcg of B_{12}
Folic acid: 800 mcg daily
Vitamin C: 100 mg twice a day
Vitamin D: 400 mg daily
Vitamin E: 400 I.U. daily
Multi-mineral tablet: 1 to 2 daily
Calcium gluconate or Bonemeal: 1000 mg daily
Iron: one tablet every three days

Type Ba

Vitamin A: 10,000 I.U. daily
Vitamin B: 1 to 3 low stress B-complex tablets daily:
$\qquad$ 5 to 10 mg of B_1
$\qquad$ 5 to 10 mg of B_2
$\qquad$ 10 mg of B_3
$\qquad$ 50 mg of B_6
$\qquad$ 100 to 500 mcg of B_{12}
Folic acid: 400 mcg daily
Vitamin C: 250 mg daily
Vitamin D: 400 mg daily
Vitamin E: 400 I.U. daily
Multi-mineral tablet: 1 to 2 daily
Calcium gluconate or Bonemeal: 500 to 700 mg daily
Glutamic acid hydrochloric: 1/2 tablet every day (or 1/8 rennet
$\qquad$ tablet)
Iron: one tablet every three days

9

CHILDREN
AND HEALTH

Being a parent is certainly a tremendous responsibility. It is also a position of considerable power. Children use their parents as models for behavior. And, without realizing it, some parents insist on very inappropriate behavior from their children. Parents train their children's taste buds. They taste the baby food before they give it to their child. If the taste does not suit them, they may add salt or sugar. Indeed, many baby foods are prepared with added salt and sugar to appeal to the taste buds of the parents. The child, then, learns to like what the parents like. Similarly, father loves baseball and buys his son a baseball hat at age six months. At two years his son has a baseball bat. The little boy learns that playing baseball is a good thing. Daddy laughs and plays with him whenever he picks up his bat. But what if the boy has Type A blood? Perhaps baseball is not a nourishing sport for his body. Perhaps, in fact, sports do not support him at all. Perhaps with his natural mental ability, he would be better nurtured if he were encouraged to read.

By recognizing the implications of our children's blood types, we can support them so that their bodies and minds will flourish. I am now treating children whose parents and grandparents have paid attention to diet according to blood type. These children have fewer health problems and are brighter, more alert, and pleasanter than any who have come to my clinic before. All children can be this healthy and vital and can develop their innate talents and gifts if their parents monitor their diet and exercise and use the clues that the child's blood type provides.

Each Child Is Different

John and Sandy are brothers. Six-year-old John is thin and wiry with blue eyes and blonde hair. Four-year-old Sandy is more solidly built, with curly brown hair and dark brown eyes. John is deeply sensitive and very bright. His teachers say he's a brilliant child. Sandy is a robust boy who loves to play baseball and ride his bicycle. He claims that he is the toughest boy at nursery school: "When somebody punches me, I punch them right back and I win." While John will spend hours drawing with pencils and paper, Sandy prefers to "zoom" his trucks around the playroom.

Though Sandy has a tendency to imitate his old brother, it is obvious that over time the two boys will develop radically different interests. John will likely be involved in intellectual and artistic pursuits, while Sandy will probably enjoy sports. Even now they have different ambitions. John wants to be an artist and Sandy wants to be a policeman. Dietary preferences are also clear already. John is not fond of meat, preferring chicken to beef. He loves vegetables and prefers fresh fruit to cookies. Sandy, on the other hand, loves hamburgers and peanut butter and hates salads. Recently their grandparents took a vacation. They came home with a gift for each child. For John, they bought a hand puppet. For Sandy they bought a toy sailboat. Each child was thrilled with his gift and neither was interested in the other's toy.

These two boys are being raised in the same family, by the same parents, and they sleep in the same room. The food available to them has been the same, and their toys are usually shared. What is different about each child, however, is his blood type. John has Type A blood and Sandy has Type O. This difference can alert their parents to their sons' uniqueness. It can guide them in determining what kind of diet, exercise, and learning environment is best for their children. If these factors are taken into account and acted on appropriately, it is likely that both children can be high achievers in school.

By checking your children's blood types, you can suit their diet and lifestyle to their own particular needs. Obviously children are not going to be divided into classrooms according to blood types. However, information about what works best for your children when learning can be shared with teachers and can certainly be implemented at home. Adjusting their diets and exercise habits to their blood type can result in academic accomplishments beyond your hopes and dreams for your children.

The Type O
Child

Type O children must use their bodies. The key to creativity and academic achievement for them is heavy physical exercise. Before class begins and intermittently throughout the day, these children should participate in vigorous physical activity. Games that involve running, such as basketball, are good for these children. When they are physically active they become more alert. Such children would be better to run and play before an examination rather than sit quietly and study. These children are "high octane children."

These children would learn best from teachers who are active and enthusiastic. Teaching methods that involve competition would be good for these children as they are highly competitive in nature. They would, for example, enjoy spelling bees. Homework assignments would be tackled with gusto, for a time. But if the child does not break after about an hour to do physical activity, she is likely to become bored and tired. Parents should remember that Type O children require physical activity.

The rooms in which these children work and play should be decorated in bright, vibrant colors. Bright oranges, yellows, and reds are suitable for Type O children. These colors resonate with their vibrant energy and will support their ability to learn.

Dietary needs include large quantities of protein, usually at two meals a day. Protein is a high-energy food, and high energy is what makes Type O children tick.

The Type A Child

These are the children of the mind. Their energy is that of the nervous system rather than of the musculo-skeletal system. Type A children love to read and quietly work by themselves. They are good at games that rely on strategy rather than endurance because their body's energy tends to come through the nervous system, Type A children are best suited to a calm environment.

If they are not given the kind of calm, quiet environment that best suits them, Type A children are likely to be hyperactive and can be mistaken for Type O's. Because their nervous systems are so sensitive, excess stimulation around them creates a frenetic response in the delicate fabric of their bodies. Their nervous systems respond to every sound and movement. These may be the children who are always busy, or who are chatterboxes or wigglers. Activity around them creates activity in their body. In order for them to use their minds effectively, they must be surrounded by calmness and peace.

Such children would flower with a teacher who spoke softly and encouraged individual work. He would work with each child individually, giving her understanding and praise. A short walk or a period of yoga or stretching exercises before classes begin would be best for Type A's. Since these children can concentrate for long periods if they are appropriately nurtured, they would not thrive on a curriculum that emphasized a variety of subjects over short periods. Rather, Type A children do best if they are assigned projects that allow them to use their intellect and creativity. Competitive games do not appeal to the Type A.

Type A children are best suited to an environment of blues and greens, the calming colors.

Because Type A children are more mental than physical, their nutritional needs are unlikely to include large amounts of protein. Lunches should be vegetarian, and dairy products should be eliminated as much as possible. Light foods allow the mind to be quick.

The Type B Child

These children experience the best of both worlds. They are in between Type O and Type A. Type B children are natural organizers. They are the children who will organize a neighbour-hood baseball game. They love to talk, to share with others. As a result they enjoy group activities. They have orderly minds and prefer an uncluttered environment. They are uncomfortable in a classroom in which desks are arranged haphazardly. They prefer a definite pattern, whether it is rows, circles, or semi-circles.

Physically, they fall between the Type A and Type O. They benefit from stretching exercises before morning classes begin and heavy physical exercise before afternoon classes. They are good at team sports. If they take up running, they are likely to do it with a friend. These children like to discuss their homework with their parents, an older sibling, or a friend.

In the classroom, Type B children benefit from group study. They do best with a teacher who has excellent communication skills and who is a group leader. This teacher would need to be orderly, presenting the children with a well thought out cirriculum. Type B children's minds operate through relationships. Thus they would want a natural order of subjects through the day. History, for example, should follow geography rather than mathematics.

Because of their innate flexibility, these children are comfortable with the full spectrum of color. Whether their room is yellow, orange, blue, or green, these children will be able to function well.

Lunches for these children should be balanced between high protein and lighter foods. Only one meal a day should contain protein.

The Type AB
Child

These children may carry traits of both Type A's and Type B's in varying quantities. To understand a Type AB child, parents should read the sections on both these blood groups. These children usually have a delicate nervous system and are often intellectual in nature. They are usually very creative, but their creativity may evidence itself in social activities, such as theater, or in individual activities, such as gymnastics.

To determine whether the A or the B is dominant, parents should examine the child carefully. Should a child suffer from mucousy conditions, have a great deal of nervous energy, and have difficulty concentrating, then he probably leans toward the A type. Recommendations for Type A's would probably be helpful here. If the child likes spending time with friends, likes to organize and mediate, and is a strategist in sports, then she probably leans toward the B type. Recommendations for Type B's may be helpful here.

These children will benefit most from stretching or yoga, and yet some may require heavy physical activity. The teacher of such children needs to be alert to the way in which their creativity and intellect are best nurtured. Some may prefer to work alone on projects while others prefer to work in groups.

Diet should lean toward lighter foods with few animal proteins and a minimum of dairy products.

Family Menus

It is not always easy to watch what our children eat. They have minds of their own (thank goodness), and as they get older, they are off by themselves more and more.

All this is complicated by the fact that there can be individuals in one family with different blood types. Where do you begin? First of all, get rid of sugars, candies, junk food, and processed foods. These are not good for anyone. Add more green vegetables, which everyone needs.

Plan menus around those items that are good for all the blood types in your family. Start with a basic that everyone can eat, and then add a little meat here for a Type O individual, and reduce eggs there for a Type A. Do the best you can.

And remember children imitate their parents. A child was brought to see me once who was asthmatic and had allergies. She was a Type A who suffered from low blood sugar. I recommended a diet of reduced carbohydrates and no candies or milk. Her condition improved quickly, but three weeks later it was worse again. On investigation, I found out that the father habitually had milk and chocolate donuts after dinner. The child, seeing her father indulge, ate them as well.

Children are a commitment. Doing what is best for them is not always easy, but it pays off in their improved health and vitality.

10

HOME
THERAPIES
FOR SPECIFIC
CONDITIONS

Many of my patients have, for some time, been trying to treat themselves in a natural way. They grow their own vegetables, shop at the health food store, eat bulgur wheat, and drink herbal teas. They take Vitamin C to combat colds. They stay away from smokers, and wear natural fibers only. Much to their dismay, they still continue to have problems. And yet they refuse to believe that they could have been doing something inappropriate for their bodies. Many people become vegetarians because they believe that it is not natural to kill animals. Their belief has nothing to do with what is natural for their body type. We cannot put our beliefs into our body and expect our body to respond. Each individual must ask "What is right for me?" Some people thrive as vegetarians, others need meat. For some people bulgur wheat is appropriate while for others soya is right.

In the following section many conditions will be discussed. Possible causes and possible treatments will be presented. Different treatments are useful to different blood types and different bodies. It is rare that I encounter a patient who has only one problem. People don't have just mirgraines or just high blood pressure; usually they have combinations of problems. A forty-eight-year-old housewife has high blood pressure, asthma, a urinary problem, and some arthritis. How she is treated depends upon the source of her problems. And treatment changes over time as conditions are alleviated. What follows are suggestions. I assume that before trying these, you have has followed the program already recommended for your blood type. If you decide to try some of the remedies, make sure, as well, that you seek the advice of a *qualified physician*.

Acne

Possible Causes: Excessive fried foods, sweets, chocolate, candies, too many dairy products, poor elimination of the bowel, stress, lack of confidence, excessive oil in the skin, hormonal changes with puberty, environment (it is not uncommon for city dwellers to move to the country and find that their acne clears up).

Treatments: Increase vegetables and roughage in the menu. Type O's should increase whole wheat and grains in the menu. Type A's should increase green vegetables. Dairy foods should be decreased. Fried foods and shellfish should be eliminated. Sweets, including all cola and sugared beverages, and chocolate should also be eliminated. Vitamin A can be increased. If there are scars on the skin, apply Vitamin E ointment or aloe vera ointment. Deodorant soaps should be eliminated. Cleanse the face three times a day with glycerine soap, alternating warm and cold water. If the skin is oily, add a pinch of salt to water, then pat on to the skin and allow to air dry. This can cause the skin to dry and result in scaling. Do not be concerned about this as it is simply old skin coming off. Hair should be washed daily. Individuals with acne should get lots of outdoor exercise — at least on hour a day. Bowel movements should occur daily. If they do not, add bran or psyllium seed or flax seed and oil to cereal in the morning. Drink at least eight glasses of water a day.

Alzheimer's Disease

Possible Causes: Years of eating badly, lack of physical exercise, premature aging, poor circulation, cholesterol build-up.

Treatments: For all blood types, all dairy products and heavy flesh foods must be eliminated for several months. Vegetables must be increased. Osteopathy, chiropractic, aromatherapy, footbaths, and colon irrigation are all essential. Extra vitamin supplementation includes lecithin, evening oil of primrose, Niacin B_6, selenium, tryptophan, Vitamin C, zinc, and magnesium. Fern phos and calcoria flour are also useful. Treatment for this condition should continue over a long period of time.

Anemia

Possible Causes: Excessive loss of blood following a heavy menstrual flow, hemmorhage, weakness in the body's ability to produce red blood cells, improper eating, iron deficiency, following a vegetarian diet when it is inappropriate for the body, lack of exercise, too much protein in the diet.

Treatments: If the reason for the anemia lies in an excessive menstrual flow, look at the hormonal system. Increase Vitamin B_6 and evening oil of primose, which would diminish excessive cramping. Increase Vitamins A, C, and E.

If hemmorhage is the cause, stop the blood flow using direct pressure. The herb aconite will reduce shock trauma. Vitamin C and rutin will speed up clotting. Iron and Vitamin B-complex may also be increased.

Inadequate production of red blood cells can be treated by increasing Vitamin B_{12}, folic acid, iron, and fern phos forum. To bring the blood back to where it should be men should take extra iron while women need to take iron and calcium.

Poor eating habits require a complete renovation of the menu. As well, the following dietary supplements should be taken: Vitamins A, B-complex, B_{12}, fern phos forum, folic acid, iron, silica, and trace minerals.

Anorexia Nervosa

Possible Causes: Emotional, underlying fatigue.

Treatments: Emotional problems should be treated by a psychologist or therapist. In order to combat fatigue, vitamin and mineral supplementation is essential. Vitamins should be ground up and given in small amounts, perhaps in oatmeal cereal. Fluids are important and must be taken. Regardless of blood type, B-complex vitamins must be given. These will help the nervous system. Acupuncture can also be useful.

Arthritis

Possible Causes: Too much flesh food and too many dairy products, poor elimination of bowels, stress, anger, faulty diet, and too little exercise.

Treatments: All blood types should reduce eggs, meat, and dairy intake as much as possible for at least three to four months to allow the uric acid to leave the joints. The number of citrus fruits eaten should be reduced, and water intake should be increased to eight glasses a day. Vitamin A should be increased and taken between meals. Make sure there are daily bowel movements by increasing the intake of green vegetables. For all blood types Vitamin C should be reduced to 250 mg a day for a period of one to two months. Calcium should be increased. Exercise is very important and must be carried out even if it hurts. A green light can be placed over affected areas for fifteen minutes daily. Rosemary steeped compresses may also be applied. Chiropractic, colon irrigation, footbaths, and aroma therapy are all beneficial. Other therapies, such as massage or acupuncture, work best once the body has been rid of toxins. It is important to remember that since arthritis normally takes many years to come about, it often takes some time to recede.

Asthma

Possible Causes: Excessive dairy intake, constipation, improper food for body type and blood type.

Treatments: Follow the diet for your blood type. Even if you are an O-type, discontinue dairy products. If that doesn't relieve the situation, discontinue wheat products. Take vitamins according to your blood type with increased amounts of Vitamins A and C as well as fern phos, lecithin, silica, and zinc. Shine a blue or green light on the chest area for fifteen minutes each day. Colon irrigations, chiropractic, and footbaths are beneficial. Many asthmatics have congested livers. A clay poultice over the liver twice a week can be helpful. Either terraxicum or dandelion teas are beneficial as well.

Blood Pressure
(High)

Possible Causes: Excessive eating, diet consisting of rich, heavy foods with large quantities of added salt resulting in a build-up of plaque along walls of the arteries, kidney problems, stress, constipation.

Treatments: Regardless of blood type, the diet must be changed dramatically. Dairy products along with heavy flesh meats like beef and pork must be eliminated. Salt must be eliminated along with foods high in sodium, such as celery or olives. Use only cold-pressed oils, such as safflower or sunflower oils. Chicken and fish may be eaten once or twice a week. Fluid intake should be increased. Eating garlic is useful as it naturally lowers blood pressure. Garlic tablets are sometimes taken.

Increased Vitamin C creates more integrity in the walls of the arteries, and rutin tablets give the walls more strength. The urinary tract can be treated with juniper berry in women and saw pometto in men. Dandelion tea is beneficial as it acts as a cleansing agent.

It is essential that the individual who has high blood pressure examines the level of stress in his life. It may be that the lifestyle needs to be altered to provide for more relaxation and quiet. Valerian tea or skull caps can be helpful in calming the body. Exercise can help, especially for those who have Type O blood, but high blood pressure is a dangerous condition and all those afflicted with it need to be supervised by a qualified physician.

Blood Pressure
(Low)

Possible Causes: Excessive work, disregard for nutritional needs of the body, genetic weakness, lack of exercise.

Treatments: O blood types should take high stress B-complex, Vitamins B_6, C, E, and A along with iron, B_{12}, folic acid, and trace minerals. If iron causes constipation, fern phos forum 6x, three tablets beneath the tongue 3 or 4 times a day can be taken.

Type A's should not take the high stress B; irons should be taken in small quantities, and Vitamin C should stay within the recommended levels for their blood type. Niacin is beneficial to all blood types because it acts as a vasodilator. Sometimes this causes flushing shortly after taking. Do not be alarmed if this happens to you. It is the vitamin working.

Bronchitis

Possible Causes: Allergies, wrong eating, lowered resistance.

Treatments: Blood types A and B should eliminate dairy products. Type O's should eliminate dairy products for a short time and then reduce severely when they return to the Type O diet. Vitamin C and Vitamin A should be increased. The menu for each blood type needs to be followed closely. A red light may be applied to the spine for 15 minutes a day and a green light to the chest for the same amount of time. Chiropractic is useful as is an inhalation of hot water and gold seal. Rosehip tea and slippery elm tea can be taken, and all supplements recommended for blood types should be taken. A day or two of rest may be necessary. Following a bout of acute bronchitis, the vitamin and mineral supplementation should continue.

Cancer

Possible Causes: I believe that natural therapies can effectively prevent cancer and other diseases that involve a breakdown in the auto-immune system. This system is damaged by improper eating and stress.

The auto-immune system is also weakened by excessive medication. Many bacteria have become resistant to medications. Medicine's response to this has been to increase the strength of antibiotics, which reduces the body's ability to heal itself. As abuse to the body increases, cells are not created at the same rate. The increased use of antibiotics may be the reason we are seeing more and more wasting diseases in our society.

The best cure for cancer is not to get it, and the best way to do that is to strengthen the body. All vitamins and minerals play an important role in the strengthening process, particularly Vitamins A, C, and B.

Take the time and effort to care for your body. You will be vastly rewarded. I have treated many patients for many years. Those who follow my programs feel revitalized and are less subject to diseases. There is much research being done by physicians into the treatment of cancer, and some people have been helped. Others have not. Cancer is more a condition to be prevented than cured.

It is important to recognize what a vital role vitamins and minerals play in our bodies and equally essential to understand what havoc sugars, carbohydrates, chemicals, and preservatives create. Nature can only balance in proportion to the abuses placed on the body.

Circulatory Problems

Phlebitis

Possible Causes: Heavy smoking, eating badly, high alcohol consumption.

Treatments: Large amounts of Vitamins C and E along with lecithin are recommended. Evening oil of primrose should also be taken. Alternate chlorophyll compresses with Vitamin E oil to affected areas. Vitamins B_6, B-complex, pantothenic acid, trace minerals, and zinc are beneficial.

While in the acute phase, refrain from standing or walking and keep legs elevated. Once the lesion begins to heal, examine your lifestyle for possible changes. Vitamins should still be taken, and exercise needs to become part of the daily routine. For Type O's, exercise needs to be integrated slowly and gradually. Type A's should start yoga and T'ai Chi along with daily walking. Leave the car at home!

Varicose Veins

Possible Causes: Childbirth, constipation, standing for long hours, sitting for long hours, crossing the knees when sitting, wearing tight garments.

Treatments: Proper bowel habits must be established. Type O's should increase their intake of fiber foods, while Type A's need to increase green vegetables. If constipation continues, add 1 tbsp. psyllium seed, 1 tbsp. flax seed, and 1 tbsp. safflower oil to cereal in the morning. Type O's should take 4 g of Vitamin C a day, while Type A's should take 1 g. Vitamin E and Vitamin A are essential.

A daily footbath consisting of two basins of water (one warm and one cold) can be useful. Alternate the feet from warm to cold to stimulate the flow of blood. If the skin on the legs is dry and flaky, one tablespoon of cold-pressed oil should be taken every day. Women who suffer from cramping of the legs should increase their calcium intake. Their needs exceed those of men. Type O's should take bonemeal or calcium orotate, while Type A's should take calcium lactate or chelated calcium. Walking is very good for varicose veins. Garments should be loose and comfortable and shoes should have low heels. Helpful therapies include footbaths, chiropractic manipulation, and light massage.

Colitis (Krohn's Disease)

Possible Causes: Stress, improper nourishment.

Treatments: All dairy products must be excluded from the diet. Type A's must adhere strictly to their menus. Type O's should exclude dairy products from their menus, should eat lean meats only, and should not consume any fried foods. Foods containing artificial additives should be removed from the diet. This means eliminating things like soft drinks, cookies, cold meats, commercial cereals, and packaged foods. Vitamins B_1, B_2, B_6, and pantothenic acid should be increased. Alfalfa tablets, digestive enzymes, garlic tablets, and okra tablets should be taken as they act on the digestive system. Drink golden seal tea two to three times a day. Chamomile tea will settle the stomach, and valerian tea is useful to relax the nervous system.

Chiropractic and foothbaths should be considered. A blue light treatment over the body can be helpful.

Constipation

Possible Causes: Eating the wrong things, especially fast foods, lack of exercise, lack of bulk in diet, not taking time to move bowels properly and regularly, inadequate water intake.

Treatments: Constipation is a disease of the cultured world. In the Third World where food consists primarily of whole grains and vegetables with only light meats, constipation is virtually unknown. Most people living in the Third World do not have automobiles. They either walk or ride bicycles.

All blood types should increase their water intake to at least eight glasses per day, but should not drink while eating. Flesh foods need to be decreased. Be sure to chew food thoroughly. Type O's need to eat more whole grains and more green vegetables and fruits. Fast foods should be eliminated. Exercise at least an hour a day. Type A's need to eat more green vegetables as well as raw salads.

Set aside a particular time in the day for a bowel movement. Stay and wait until you are successful. You are teaching the body. Above all, be patient. Retraining takes time.

Eczema/
Psoriasis/
Allergies

Possible Causes: Faulty elimination of bowel. If there is poor elimination of the bowel and toxins cannot be eliminated through the kidneys, then the next organ available for elimination is the skin.

Treatments: To reverse such conditions, the body must be cleansed and given a proper diet. All blood types should follow recommended menus. Type O's should temporarily stop eating dairy and flesh foods. After the body is cleansed, these things can be re-introduced. Type A's should stay away from all dairy and flesh food permanently. Colon irrigation, foothbaths, and chiropractic manipulation are needed to cleanse the body. The liver should be cleaned with dandelion tea. Vitamins A and E are especially important.

Eye Conditions

Possible Causes: Pollution, chemical irritants, fluorescent lighting, sugar.

Treatments: Ideally, one should remove himself from the environmental source of the difficulty. This is, of course, not always possible. As much as possible, fluorescent lighting should be changed to incandescent or full spectrum lighting. Studies in factories and schools show that workers are more productive and children retain information better if lighting is incandescent or full spectrum rather than fluorescent. The best of all lights, however, is sunlight.

Individuals who have any eye condition should always live in homes that have lots of sunlight. Those with cataracts should remove sugars and starches from their diets. Individuals with glaucoma are wise to eliminate dairy products and red meats. Vitamin A should always be taken by people who suffer from eye conditions. Those with cataracts may find golden seal compresses to the eye helpful. Glaucoma patients should remove salt from the diet and increase their daily intake of water.

For those who require glasses, Dr. Bates has developed eye exercises which, if done for five to ten minutes, two to three times a day, can improve vision markedly. Hold a pencil at arm's length and focus on the eraser. Move the pencil clockwise, then counter-clockwise, always keeping the pencil at the periphery of your vision. Do not turn your head. Keep focusing on the eraser. Alternate eyes. These exercises will strengthen the eye muscles and will assist the lenses. Remove your glasses for half an hour each day, increasing the time as your vision improves.

Remember, above all, work in sunlight as much as possible. Bookkeepers, accountants, and others who do work that requires excessive use of the eyes should ensure their desks get enough light.

Gall Bladder Problems

Probable Causes: Improper eating, rich food, heavy meat, greasy, fried foods, overeating, obesity, stress, lack of exercise.

Possible Treatments: Following improper eating habits, the gall bladder secretes bile to cleanse the body and break down fats (bile is an emulsifier). To correct gall bladder problems, all fats must be reduced in the diet. Colon irrigation, footbaths, chiropractic, acupuncture, aromatherapy, and clay packs are all useful. All morid matter must be removed from the body. A lesser type of protein food, like cheese or tofu, should then be eaten with plenty of green vegetables and grains. Follow the vitamin list for your blood type closely. Evening oil of primose should be increased, and lecithin, enzymes, and bile salts should be taken following meals. China off 6x, chionath, and calclus 1/8-10x are homeopathic remedies that can be helpful.

Gout

Possible Causes: Improper eating. (This illness occurs in all blood types when too many animal products have been eaten over long periods of time. Years ago it was a disease of the rich.)

Possible Treatments: Stick closely to the menus for your blood type. Type O's should also reduce flesh foods for about six months. Fluid intake should include 8 to 12 glasses of water every day. Vitamin B_6, B_{12}, evening oil of primrose, and lecithin along with Vitamin E should be increased. Colon irrigations and footbaths are essential. Homeopathic herbs can include amm benz, calchi, ferr phos 6x, fornica, fraximus, lidum, lithium, ly cop, natrim phos 6x, or urtica.

Heart Conditions

Possible Causes: Stress, abusive eating (heavy, rich foods), inadequate exercise.

Treatments: In many respects, what is required is a total shift in values in relation to food, work, stress, and physical exercise. All blood types need to remove fats from their diets as well as reduce protein intake. A-types should become strict vegetarians and remove all dairy products from their diets. All types should eat more fruit. Supplements for blood types should be amplified in the following ways: Vitamins B, C, and E should be Lecithin and evening oil of primose can be added. Lecithin cleans the blood vessels, and evening oil of primrose reduces plaque build-up. If blood pressure is high, rutin should be included. Herbal additions should include hawthorn berry, cratalgus, and plenty of herbal teas. Garlic should be added to the diet. Chiropractic, colon irrigation, acupuncture, and light massage are all useful in correcting heart conditions.

One other hint: If you life in a cold climate, do not vacation in a hot climate for a week and then return. This creates a severe stress on the cardiovascular system. In a cold climate, an individual's blood is more viscous than in a warm climate. The blood thins out in a hot climate. If an individual goes to a hot climate for a short time and quickly returns, the blood has to adapt twice, once to the heat and once to the cold. This change is very hard on the body.

Hypoglycemia

Probable Causes: Hypoglycemia seems to be the disease of the day. About 65 percent of people in North America between the ages of three and forty have some form of sugar intolerance caused by the consumption of quantities of refined foods. Vast amounts of carbohydrates and chemicals are being eaten. Many of us are, in a sense, addicted to these foods. Their excess consumption results in our feeling tired when we awake in the morning after a good night's sleep. After lunch we want a twenty minute nap. In the middle of the afternoon we are exhausted. If we examine the foods we normally eat, we find that two-thirds of our diet consists of sugar and starch in the form of potatoes, rice, bread, and even some fruits and vegetables! Sugar intolerances of any severity are debilitating to our quality of life. We cannot experience our full potential while addicted to sugars and carbohydrates. As a result, we fail to make the contribution we could in life.

Treatments: Breaking the sugar/carbohydrate habit is arduous. To begin with, our palates have become accustomed to carbohydrates. Many of us do not feel replete after a meal unless we complete it with something sweet. The five to seven weeks it takes to "kick the sugar habit" are as difficult a time as anyone can spend. It is essential to be committed to this shift in diet, and it is usually easiest done when someone is available for support. Here are the rules:

1. *No soft drinks, alcohol, sugar, honey or molasses.*

2. *Bread must be reduced to half or one slice a day.*

3. *Potato must be replaced with a quarter cup brown rice per day.*

A daily menu would look like this:

On rising, drink the juice of half a lemon in a glass of water. O and B blood types should then exercise for twenty minutes. Type A's should do yoga. Following the exercise an energy drink should be taken. For Types O and B this consists of:

    1 tbsp. soya powder
    2 tbsp. lecithin granules
    1 thsp. yeast
    1 tbsp. liquid protein
    4 to 5 oz. water

Type A's take the same drink, but eliminate the yeast.
    For breakfast Types O and B can have

    1/2 grapefruit
    1/2 cup cooked cereal with skim milk, or one egg
    herbal tea
    vitamins

Type A's can have health food store cereal, like puffed rice, with soymilk. Two or three days a week they may substitute an egg for the cereal.

Lunch should consist of a salad of six or seven vegetables, tofu, herbal tea, and vitamins.

The three o'clock snack can consist of almonds and sunflower seeds.

At six, eat a meal of fish or chicken and at least five vegetables for all blood types. (Type A's cannot tolerate a vegetarian diet until the sugar intolerance is cured.)

Vitamins should also be taken by all blood types. Note that the daily vitamin regimen should include increased B-complex, niacin, B_6, zinc, chromium, selenium, iron, and Vitamin C.

It may take up to six months of a strict diet before you begin to experience your energetic and enthusiastic self. It may take one or two years before you are no longer addicted.

Insomnia

Probable Causes: Stress, frequent changes of sleep patterns (shift work), inadequate Vitamin B-complex, poor ventilation, hormonal imbalances.

Possible Treatments: Sleep is necessary for life. While we sleep the body regenerates and repairs itself. During they alpha, or dream, state most repair occurs. If you follow the supplements for your blood type closely, it is unlikely that vitamin deficiency is a cause of your sleeping problem. Increase the ventilation in your home and work place. If you are under a great deal of stress, 600 mg of tryptophen taken one hour before bedtime can be helpful. Increasing the intake of calcium may also help, as might valerian tea at bedtime.

Liver Ailments

Probable Causes: Improper nutrition, infection, large amounts of medication, especially antibiotics.

Possible Treatments: The liver is the largest organ of the body, and yet it is little understood. Its main function is to filter waste and metabolize chemicals. After years of abuse from chemicals like alcohol or from repeated doses of medication, it becomes sluggish and diseased. Jaundice can develop. Castor oil or clay packs can be used as a treatment.

Place a piece of plastic underneath the body while the treatment is being carried on. Soak a cloth in castor oil. Place the cloth over the liver (right rib cage to the sternum, down to the belly button and across over to the right hip bone). Place a hot-water bottle containing lukewarm tap-water over the cloth and keep in place for half to three-quarters of an hour.

All blood types should follow their menus scrupulously and take recommended supplements. Vitamin B-complex, vitamin B_{12} and folic acid should be increased. Colon irrigation, foothbaths, chiropractic, and clay packs should be done. Homeopathic remedies include natrim phos, kali pic, bry chin, cholist, and kali myrica.

Low Back Pain

Possible Causes: Overextension of the body either in work or play can cause pain. If there is a misalignment of the vertebrae, the individual may end up with chronic pain. Constipation and hormonal imbalances can also cause pain.

Treatments: Calcium, Vitamin C, and minerals should be increased. Herbs rhus toricodendron and anica mont can help. Apply moist compresses or run a hot shower on the lower back. Acupuncture, chiropractic, and shiatsu are all very effective treatments for low back pain. Dairy products and heavy meats should be reduced to a minimum. Colon irrigation can also improve back conditions.

Migraine

Possible Causes: Stress, misalignment of spinal curvature, constipation, poor elimination, abusive food, trauma.

Treatments: To begin with, it is essential that the diet be changed. Fried foods must be given up, and the blood type menu should be followed closely. Colon irrigation and footbaths are recommended even if there is proper elimination. Chiropractic manipulation is also helpful. Coffee, alcohol, and smoking must be eliminated. These three items reduce oxygen flow to the brain. Calcium should be added to supplements, and pantothenic acid, niacin, Vitamin C, Vitamin B_6, and trace minerals should be increased. Linden tea compresses to the nape of the neck are helpful.

Neuritis

Possible Causes: Whether trigeminal neuralgia or numbness of the extremities, neuritis is usually caused by trauma, missalignment of the spine or lack of Vitamin B-complex.

Treatments: Chiropractic manipulation is very important, especially for vertebral misalignment. Supplements should include increased amounts of Vitamin B$_6$, pantothenic acid, niacin, and calcium. Women need more calcium than men, and the type should be chosen according to blood type. If the neuritis is in the shoulder or neck area, a linden tea poultice applied to the area for 15 to 20 minutes twice a day can be helpful. (To make this poultice steep five tablespoons of tea in five cups of boiling water for 10 minutes. Strain the tea and place a cloth in the strained water. Apply to affected area.) Other helpful herbs are rhus toricodendron and anica mont. Increased fluid intake is also important.

Prostate Conditions

Possible Causes: Improper eating, especially too many rich foods with heavy gravy and spices, too much or a lack of sexual activity, kidney or bladder irritations or infections.

Treatments: Follow the menu for your blood type and increase foods from the vegetable kingdom. Remove alcoholic beverages, coffee, tea, and spices from your diet, and drink six to eight glasses of water every day. Horsetail tea is good to drink. Boil a handful of parsley in water for three-quarters of an hour and drink one cup every day. Follow blood type supplements and increase the amount of zinc, magnesium, Vitamin B$_6$, Vitamin C, and Vitamin A. Diathermy and sitz baths are helpful. Soak in a bathtub of lukewarm water with three tablespoons of epsom salts once a day.

Sore Throats/Sinus Conditions

Possible Causes: The most common cause of both conditions is improper diet, which can result in postnasal drip or phlegm in the back of the throat on rising.

Treatments: Dairy products should be eliminated from all blood types until symptoms have passed. If the problem recurs, there maybe some leaning toward the A-type, and dairy products should be reduced permanently. For relief of immediate symptoms, a carrot poultice (grated carrot in white cloth) can be wrapped around the neck. For nasal drip, inhale lukewarm water in which a pinch of salt has been dissolved.

One other reason for colds in winter is overheating of bedrooms at night. The dryness of the air causes mucous membranes to dry up. The window should always be partly open in winter and a vaporizer should be running in the bedroom at all times.

Ulcers

Possible Causes: Stress, wrong eating.

Treatments: Figure out which areas in your life are causing stress and resolve as many of them as you are willing to. Greasy foods must be given up, and milk should be avoided. These make ulcers worse. Raw cabbage juice from a blender is very good for ulcers. Extra enzymes should also be taken. Digestive herbal teas, such as golden seal, are helpful. During episodes of pain, cook oatmeal in water then squeeze through a cheesecloth. Reserve the water and mix it in equal parts with soy milk. Drink one cup at a time. Colon irrigation, chiropractic, acupuncture, and massage all help this condition.

Urinary Tract
Ailments

Possible Causes: Improper eating, lack of proper fluids, alcohol abuse, excessive dairy or flesh intake.

Possible Treatments: Proper foods must be eaten. If kidney stones form out of uric acid, meat intake should be reduced dramatically. If kidney stones form out of calcium oxilate, calcium intake must be decreased. Eight to twelve glasses of water must be drunk daily. Pantothenic acid, Vitamins C, A, and B_6 should also be increased.

11

CANDIDA OR
YEAST

Yeast has interested me for many years. Lately, more and more people are also looking at it and its effects on our health. Yeast in and of itself is not a bacteria; it is almost plant-like in origin and is found in the majority of the food we eat and in the air we breath. It is found in bread, juice, jam, chocolate, noodles, cakes, candies, beer, wine, cheeses, mushrooms, and certain vitamins.

After we have eaten yeast and yeast products for years, the yeast begins to colonize in our intestinal tracts. Then by eating other foods, such as sugars and starches, we allow the yeast to grow and spread. What actually happens is that once the yeast is colonized in our digestive systems then the eating of carbohydrates gives the yeast a base to feed upon.

How many of us, while drying ourselves after our morning shower, look in the mirror and see how flat our tummies are, only to notice that during the day our abdomens distend. By the end of the evening we need to loosen our waistbands because of the bloating. This is yeast. All day long, what we eat feeds the yeast. The yeast tends to create gas and that in turn causes the bloatedness. Just as yeast causes bread dough to rise so it causes the distention in the abdomen.

Yeast also has an effect on the mind. It can cause us to become irritable and depressed. People may suffer from headaches, anxiety, and mood changes — happy one minute and then, for no apparent reason, moody the next.

Getting Rid of Yeast

To rid yourself of the yeast condition and its effects, you need a very strong mental attitude. It is not a condition that will clear up in a matter of days or weeks. Your body may take up to nine months to divest itself of the condition. The stronger position you take in the beginning, the more likely that you are to be successful. Just remember that it is only for a short period out of your whole lifetime. Until you once again experience abundant health and mental clarity, it is important that you follow your diet carefully.

It is important first of all to refrain from feeding the existing yeast. To do that, avoid putting sugars or starches, which will become a sugar, into your body. Breads that have yeast need to be eliminated in favor of sprouted breads and non-yeast bread. You can buy sprouted breads or breads with no yeast in a health food store. Some supermarkets sell a sour-dough yeast-free bread. Check your cereal boxes and other labels to see that the products contain no sugar and no yeast. Eliminate juices and fruits, wines and sodas, mushrooms, cakes, candies, potatoes, macaroni, rice.

If it seems that I am saying that you should eliminate eating altogether, do not despair: there are plenty of products that have no yeast in them — including most of the vegetable kingdom, soya products, and soya breads. Many cereals are yeast-free, as are poultry, meats, and fish.

The body needs some carbohydrates. What you don't want to do is eat a carbohydrate that has yeast. Instead, monitor the amount of carbohydrate you are putting into your body. In place of your usual three slices of bread, have one slice of yeast-free bread. Instead of a large bowl of cereal in the morning for breakfast, have a half bowl of yeast-free cereal. Instead of white rice or potatoes, eat brown rice. While the brown rice converts into a sugar that supports the yeast, the breakdown occurs very slowly in the body, whereas the white rice and potatoes convert into a sugar the moment they meet with the salivary glands.

Women who have recurring vaginal discharges may be helped by a douche of one cup of cool golden seal tea mixed with about five tablespoons of yogurt. This can be used once or twice a day by all blood types. Yeast frequently also affects women's hormonal systems and creates irregular menstrual flows. If the condition remains within the body, it eventually affects the urinary tract, and some women may develop cystitis and other urinary tract irritations.

It is also important to destroy the existing yeast. You can do this in many ways. Yogurt is a good treatment for O and B blood types, but not for Type A because its dairy base tends to create mucous. Caprylic acid is very beneficial in destroying yeast and can be obtained from health food stores. Caprylic acid is a refined acid olive oil molecule and doesn't kill the yeast but interferes with the budding. Homoeopathic tinctures of candida are also beneficial as is garlic. Garlic an be taken in its natural form or in tablets. Deodorized garlic, in my opinion, has little or no effect, although garlic with parsley would be very helpful — both for the candida and for keeping your friends! These last three items can be taken by all blood types.

Once you begin to eliminate the yeast from your body, you can expect to experience fatigue, emotional swings, diarrhea, and other upsets for about two weeks, but these do go away. Soon you will awaken in the morning full of energy and health, without aches and pains, and with more mental clarity.

You must, however, continue to be careful with yeast products. A periodic dousing with a natural substance that interferes with or kills the yeast may be the answer. Once you have gotten the deep-seated yeast out of your body, your urinary tract, and your digestive system, you can periodically eat yeast. Then, maybe every two or three months, you will need to take caprylic acid for three or four days to keep everything in control. You'll need to experiment. For Type O's a three or four day dousing of caprylic acid may be beneficial every six months to once a year. For Type B, every six months is better, and if for Types A or AB, maybe every three months.

As with this and all illnesses, discuss your symptoms and ailments with your physician.

12

CHILDREN'S
DISEASES

When you become a parent, you take on an awesome responsibility. The child that has come through you into the world has his own mind and its own destiny. You need to guide him with love and positive support. You need to be conscious of your actions since your children will copy them. If you smoke, your children are likely to smoke. If you eat red meat every day and drink a glass of milk with every meal, your children are likely to do the same. If you eat candies when you are upset, your children will do the same. If you are angry, your children will be, too. Children want to be loved and will do whatever they can to please. If sickness brings them the attention they crave, they will learn to be sick. Sickness can be something a child learns.

Almost 90 percent of children's diseases can be prevented. Most are caused by poor nutritional patterns or by emotional upsets. If children are kept away from high carbohydrate foods and sugar, if their rooms are ventilated at night, if they get adequate exercise and rest, if they are given proper vitamins, if they eat according to blood types, and if they are given emotional security, they will thrive.

The most common complaints of children are stomach aches and colds. Stomach aches are usually caused by sluggish bowels (which are caused by inadequate nutrition or lack of exercise). Most cold are caused by overexertion and poor nutrition.

Fever

Fevers of 100 to 102°F are not to be considered dangerous in children. The raised temperature simply indicates that the body's immune system is rallying. If a child has an infection, the hypothalamus produces a fever to allow the blood to circulate faster, bringing antibodies in the blood to affected areas to envelop the bacteria. When we give our children ASA to combat a fever, we slow down the flow of blood and the antibodies do not reach affected areas quickly. Bacteria are thus allowed to spread more quickly. It is important to recognize that low-grade fevers can be helpful to the child.

Probable Cause: Fevers that are not accompanied by other symptoms are probably related to the ingestion of junk food. High carbohydrate and sweet foods produce large amounts of morbid material in the digestive system. Until this has been excreted, the child may have a fever.

Possible Treatment: With correct supervision from a professional, one or two enemas may be enough to reduce the fever. I cannot overemphasize the importance of cleaning the bowel. In addition, the child should be given plenty of liquid. The body must not be allowed to dehydrate. Homeopathic fern phos 6x under the tongue can also be helpful. Vitamin C and echanasia C can be given for cold and flu symptoms. Golden seal tea, chamomile tea, or homeopathic nox vomica can be useful for stomach distress.

Common Colds

Possible Causes: One of the main reasons children get colds is that their rooms are not ventilated properly. At night, parents close the windows and the door to the room. In winter the room becomes hot and stuffy. This situation results in headaches and head colds. The combination of dry air and increased carbon dioxide over the night creates the perfect environment for colds. Of course, another contributing factor is the ingestion of large quantities of junk food and excess dairy products. These foods increase quantities of mucous in the body and result in clogging the system.

Possible Treatment: To begin with, as a prevention, windows and doors should be left open at night. A humidifier in the room is also helpful. All blood types should be given increased quantities of Vitamin C — preferably with echanasia — and Vitamin A. If the cold is in the bronchial tree, take the child into the bathroom and turn on the hot water to create steam. This will assist breathing. A vaporizer with eucalyptus oil added can also help. The head of the bed should be raised 4 to 5 inches. It is important that the child drink lots of fluids and that his bowels are kept open. If the child is coughing but has no phlegm, use a mustard plaster. (To make a mustard plaster, mix one cup of flour with two tablespoons of dried mustard. Make a hole in the centre of the mixture and pour in enough hot water to make a paste. Spread the paste on a cotton dish towel and put the plaster on the child's chest. *The cloth surface, not the paste, should rest on the child's skin. Otherwise, burns can occur.* The child *must* be under the covers before, during, and after the application of a mustard plaster. The plaster goes on the front of the chest until the child can feel the heat (about three or four minutes). The child should then lie on his stomach and the plaster can be applied to the back for another three to four minutes. An adult should stay with a child during the application of the plaster. Never use a plaster on an infant.

Following the removal of the plaster, give the child a cup of strong rosehip tea with one tablespoon of honey and one tablespoon of brandy. She should remain in bed and under the sheets. Sweating may occur and pajamas and bedclothes may need to be changed. Vitamin C should be taken every two hours throughout the day.

Sore Throats

Possible Cause: Improper diet, post-nasal drip, tonsillitis

Possible Treatments: Grate a raw carrot and put in a cotton cloth. Fold the cloth over and wrap around the throat for 15 to 20 minutes twice a day. An alternative is to prepare a cabbage poultice in the same way you prepare a carrot poultice. Salt and water or a solution of two-thirds water and one-third vinegar can be gargled. Vitamin C and Vitamin A should be taken every two hours.

Children suffer from sore throats and sinus trouble frequently. Far and away the most common cause of children's colds are improper eating and improper elimination. Has the child recently eaten a lot of junk food or unusually large amounts of dairy products? Is he eliminating frequently and evacuating completely?

Tonsillitis

Many years ago, inflamed tonsils were automatically removed. It was believed that they had no value. We now know that they are the protectors of the sinus and throat. Parents should do everything possible to avoid surgery. Seek the advice of a physician whose leanings are toward natural therapies. Increasing intake of Vitamin C, especially Vitamin C with echanasia, is very helpful. There are many homeopathic remedies available, such as glycothalmaline gargle or vita laca bayberry, but these should be given under supervision of a qualified physician. Glycothalmaline gargles, carrot and cabbage poultices, and tea tree oil mists can be helpful. Regardless of blood type, dairy products should be reduced.

Asthma

Possible Causes: Improper diet

Possible Treatments: Asthma is a condition which tells us that waste products are not being eliminated properly through the kidneys and the bowel. Instead, the body discards them through the lungs. It is thus essential that the bowels are eliminating completely and that the kidneys are being flushed with water. It is essential that the child drink large quantities of water, preferably eight to ten glasses daily. If a child refuses to take water, fruit juice can be given, but it should be well diluted with water.

Regardless of blood type, all dairy products should be removed from the diet. Substitute soya milk for whole milk and avoid cheese. Extra vitamins will strengthen the immune system. The child should also eat lots of green vegetables.

There are many homeopathic herbs available for asthmatic conditions, but these must be monitored by a physician.

Stomach Aches

Possible Causes: Improper elimination of the bowel, tension, wrong combination of foods

Possible Treatment: It is often difficult for parents to imagine that tension could enter their child's world. Children do not need to meet mortgage payments and do not have concerns about a career. However, children do participate in a society of other children. What looks like a minor disappointment to a parent can feel like a major catastrophe to a child. Such upsets can affect the digestive system. Often, a stomach ache will go away if a parent spends some quiet time with the child and talks to him about his upset.

The parent should also check on the foods the child has been eating. If he has eaten lots of sweets or foods that are new to his system. he may feel ill. Do not let the child eat anything for a while, but do give him frequent small quantities of water. Golden seal tea is very helpful, one tablespoon at a time. Always treat stomach conditions with bitters, not sweets. Slippery elm and dandelion teas are also good.

If the child has not moved his bowels for a few days, he may also develop a stomach ache. An enema may be the treatment of choice. However, *never give a child who has a stomach ache an enema until a qualified physician has ruled out appendicitis.*

Finally, if the stomach ache persists for longer than one day, the child should see a physician.

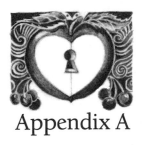

Appendix A

DIAGNOSTIC PROCEDURES

When diagnosing, I use three tools: iridology, pulse diagnosis, and blood typing. Diagnosis is actually an interplay between these three methods. By taking the pulses first, I get a general idea of possible weaknesses. Blood typing usually affirms my findings and allows me to focus my attention. Iridology validates the other two. I then can come to concrete decisions about what produces symptoms and what specific menu, exercise plan, supplements, and therapies will reverse known conditions.

Iridology

By examining the iris of the eye we are able to see all the weaknesses an individual has produced in his body since birth. It is as if the iris is the recorder for the body. On the accompanying diagram you will see landmarks identified. Each landmark corresponds with specific areas of the body. The eye is zonal. The 12 o'clock position represents one area (the head), while another position, say, 6 o'clock represents another (the foot). By bringing your eye close to a mirror and then shining a flashlight onto the mirror, you will see various markings on the iris. There may be black spots, or white circles. The markings indicate various weaknesses in the body.

The first inner circle represents the sympathetic and parasympathetic nervous systems. Jutting out from this circle may be stress lines. If they are fine speckles, the individual has a tendency to hold stress within the body; his temper is never let out. If the speckling is placed inside the circle as well as on the rest of the iris, the individual releases tension through temper tantrums.

There are other circles in the eyes. These I call rings of toxicity. Zero is perfection while five is the highest level possible. One in 800 people will have five rings of toxicity. These can be reduced as eating habits are improved and as colon irrigations are taken. As the rings disappear, fewer and fewer colon irrigations are needed.

Mucous clots are little round yellowish or whitish clumps on the retina close to the circulatory system ring. Sometimes they are so severe they reach the nervous system. This means that the individual has overburdened her body with dairy products. If such spots are seen, dairy products should be eliminated from the diet regardless of blood type until the condition is removed from the body. If this warning is ignored, high blood pressure, clogged arteries, frequent colds, cold feet, cold hands, dizziness, or lapses in memory can occur.

Acute conditions in the body appear as a whiteness with a little yellow. If such a mark appears, for example, in the area identified as sinuses, the individual probably has daily sinus attacks. As therapy is taken, the white turns to gray and the condition is no longer acute. It is going into check. Eventually it will become black as the condition leaves, and the iris will return to its original colour.

If there is a dark elliptical mark on the iris, there has been a condition in the past which was resolved. If the outside of the mark has white superimposed over it, the condition has once again become acute. Conditions that are genetic in origin also appear as dark spots. These will take some time to resolve. If a person has a problem with the adrenals, he may be under great strain or he may have arthritis. If he also shows a weakness in the pancreas, he probably has hypoglycemia. If there is only a weakness in the pancreas, then he probably has diabetes. A mark in the liver area

Dr. D'Adamo's Iridology Chart

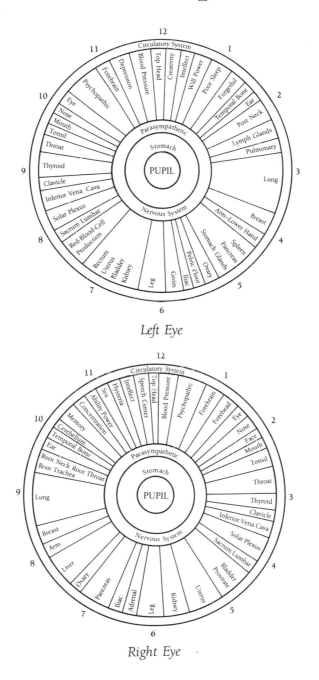

Left Eye

Right Eye

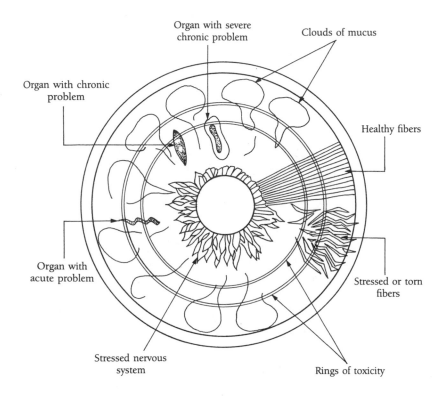

may mean that at one time an individual was taking large doses of medication. If this intake of drugs went on for a very long time, it is possible that the spleen will show a weakness. However, a splenic weakness may mean that an individual had mononucleosis at one time. Lung plus kidney weaknesses usually mean asthma.

It takes some time to be able to read the iris well. However, looking at the landmarks closely and putting them together with any symptoms you may have, may give some clue to your body's weaknesses.

Pulse diagnosis

When I talk about the pulses, I do not mean the pulse that physician takes. Nor do I mean the oriental pulses. The pulse is taken with three fingers, the thumb should be on the back of the wrist. The following diagrams indicate what each pulse means.

Right Hand

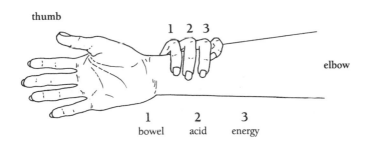

thumb

1　2　3

elbow

1	2	3
bowel	acid	energy

1	2	3
gall bladder	small intestines	kidney
liver		

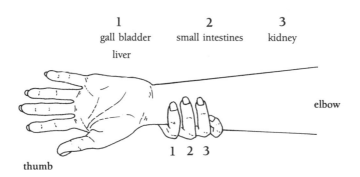

elbow

1　2　3

thumb

Left Hand

Each area is checked by each finger. If the finger that lies over energy feels a feeble beat compared to the others, there is an indication of fatigue. If it is really feeble, exhaustion is probably present. Blood may also be circulating poorly.

With the middle pulse, if the beat is high, the acid level is probably high. If it is low, the acid level is probably low. It is likely that an A blood type will have hypoacidity, and an O blood type will have hyperacidity.

With the last pulse, a slow sluggish beat will indicate poor evacuation of the bowel and possibly constipation. A very strong pulse will indicate diarrhea or colitis. On some occasions, however, a low, thready pulse will indicate colitis. Again, evacuation is not proper even if diarrhea seems to be present. Nature is trying to cleanse the bowel.

On the left side, the finger that tests the kidney pulse may find a weak pulse. This indicates improper fluid intake or a possible kidney or bladder problem.

The middle pulse reflects the functioning of the small intestine. If there is a low pulse, food is fermenting in the small intestine. If the pulse is high, the individual tends not to chew his food properly. He is probably a gulper. If the pulse is thready, the food is not broken down properly.

The last pulse measures the gall bladder and liver. We discover how well the bile is emulsifying fats. If the pulse is very high, the gall bladder is under strain.

Pulse diagnosis is actually rather complicated and takes many months to learn.

Appendix B

CLEANSING
THERAPIES

Why are
Therapies
Necessary?

Eating a proper diet, getting appropriate exercise, and taking needed supplements are all essential to achieve and maintain vibrant, vital health. To reverse limiting conditions and cure chronic ailments cleansing therapies are often requrired as well. After years of improper eating and inadequate exercise, most adult bodies have become toxic. Substances such as uric acid and mucous have accumulated in tissues and organs. This collection of abnormal waste materials within the body is one of the main reasons for the deteriorating condition most of us experience with age. In order to get maximum benefit from diet, exercise, and supplements, toxic substances must be removed.

Toxic substances collect in all parts of the body if they are not excreted properly. An individual who eats large amounts of mucous-forming foods such as dairy products and fatty meats, without balancing them with whole-grain products, ample vegetables, many different fruits, and adequate exercise, will slow down the elimination process in the bowel. If this same person avoids exercise and does not drink enough water, natural muscle action and lubrication will be considerably reduced, and a lot of waste material will remain in the bowel. The musculature designed to move the material through is not strong enough to combat the collections of mucous, impacted matter, and dead bacteria. The bowel is designed to absorb any nutrients left after the small intestine has done its work. If waste material collects in the colon long enough, the body begins to absorb toxins rather than nutrients because that is all available to it.

Similarly, the kidneys can become overburdened and not do the job they are supposed to do. They act as a filtration system, sifting out uric acid and other substances from the bloodstream. If the kidneys have to work overtime to clean the blood, they will reduce their functioning. Toxic substances end up circulating in the blood and are deposited in cells and tissues. Weaknesses in the lungs, kidneys, liver, heart, circulatory system, prostate gland, and pancreas along with a variety of aches and pains may result.

Similarly, an overworked liver will break down, further hampering the kidneys, and ultimately causing waste matter to be deposited in cells. Cell oxidation is then threatened. When cells do not get enough oxygen, biochemical processes are altered, and the body becomes susceptible to many different diseases.

If we do not exercise properly, our muscles become either taut, in which case they require stretching, or weak, and in need of toning. When our muscles are not strong and supple, they place considerable strain on our bones, notably the spinal column. The spinal column is the guardian of the central nervous system and is held in place by our muscles. If we are out of shape physically, the vertebrae are liable to move out of place, causing enervation of all our major organs. Messages sent from the brain may be improperly received by our organs. For example, the heart muscle may not contract as strongly as it normally does because a thoracic vertebrae has shifted position, slightly blocking a message being sent through it to our strongest muscle. If this happens repeatedly, blood flow through the heart may be reduced. This condition could, of course, result in many possible complications.

There are many therapies available to correct illnesses that occur as a result of our poor habits. Colons can be emptied, kidneys can be cleansed, and vertebrae can be put in place. Such therapies work hand in hand with proper diet, exercise, and supplementation. Proper foods will assure the body of adequate nutrition. Proper exercise will keep muscles strong and promote oxygenation of the cells. It increases muscle tone and improves cardiac functioning as well as general circulation. Supplementation will strengthen weakened cells so that adjustments made through therapies will remain permanently.

The natural therapies discussed here should be undertaken under the advice of a qualified physician.

Acupuncture

Acupuncture dates back some 5,000 years. The principles behind this therapy are that within the body are 12 meridians, that must be balanced for the body to be healthy. The acupuncturist uses needles or an electronic acupuncture machine to affect the meridians and to balance one with another. For thousands of years this was the poor man's medicine in China. Following Mao Tse Tung's rule, it began to be practiced openly. Acupuncture has become an integral part of western natural healing.

Aromatherapy

Aromatherapy is a gentle massage that introduces essential oils to the body. Applied to the skin, these oils produce either a calming or a stimulating effect, depending on the oil used. Thus, neuromuscular systems can be affected. Some oils also drain the lymphatic system, the body's natural cleansing system. In combination with other therapies, aromatherapy is very beneficial.

Chiropractic Manipulation

Chiropractic manipulation has been used for hundreds of years, but it is only in the last 25 to 30 years that it has been given its rightful place in the healing arts. Chiropractic focuses on the vertebral column, which houses the nervous system. Because of the stress and strain of life, vertebra frequently impinge on the spinal cord, thus affecting nerve supply to vital organs. When messages from the nervous system are not properly conveyed to parts of the body, illness results. The chiropractor locates any misalignments and manually manipulates the vertabra, returning it to its natural position and re-establishing normal nerve supply to the affected areas. Chiropractic is one of the most important of all the natural therapies, for without proper nerve supply the human body cannot remain healthy.

Colon Irrigation

About 98 percent of all patients who come to me require a series of colon irrigations. The colons of most people have collected large amounts of waste material over the years. These accumulations cause a build-up of compacted waste matter on the wall of the bowel. Three things happen when waste collects in this way. First, it blocks the blood corpuscles that line the wall of the colon, preventing the vital nutrients in recently consumed material from being extracted and placed into the bloodstream. Thus, any possible nutritive value to the body is blocked. Second, after a period of time the compacted waste ferments, decays, and putrefies so that what is available to the body to absorb are large amounts of dead bacteria, acid, and other toxins. One quarter to one half of the organic matter in fecal material has been found to be made up of living and dead bacteria. Eventually these toxins are absorbed from the large intestine and are normally excreted in the urine. There is considerable evidence to demonstrate that these toxins are far more dangerous than previously believed. If they are given either orally or intravenously they have been found to be powerful poisons. Third, as waste material collects in the colon, it stretches and weakens the natural musculature so that proper evacuation cannot occur. Thus, more and more waste collects.

These problems usually originate with improper eating and improper exercise. Unfortunately, even reverting to proper exercise and diet will not resolve the problem. Because musculature is weakened and colon walls are coated, the body still cannot absorb the nutrients. Colon irrigation will remove debris from the walls and allow cells to function properly.

Eliminating every day does not necessarily imply that waste materials are not collecting in the colon. Eliminated material should come close to the amount eaten in a day. Even a small amount left behind will cause problems. Women, especially, may notice that the upper part of their abdomen is flat while the lower part is bloated. Impacted material in the transverse colon stretches and causes the colon to dip. Muscles flex and drop down in the abdomen compounding constipation problems.

Many physicians take a dim view of colon irrigation. They think it (1) depletes the body of natural salts; (2) destroys normal flora; (3) leaves one dependant on irrigations for elimination; and, (4) spreads bacteria. None of these need to happen. If it is done under the auspices of a qualified physician with appropriate hygenic precautions being taken, colon irrigation replaces salts and flora and does not cause dependancy.

This therapy is not invasive. The colon is merely washed with warm water. No force to insert the water or suction to remove it is required. Gravity provides everything that is needed for a successful irrigation. Results can be remarkable. I have treated individuals who in the past had poor bowel habits, perhaps evacuating every two or three days, instead of daily. Since they were absorbing toxins into their bloodstream, they experienced lethargy, mild depression, poor humor, and inability to concentrate. After the bowel was evacuated, all these symptoms were eliminated. Indeed, 600 years ago Maimonedes noted that if the bowels do not move completely, the mind becomes tense and nervous. If the condition continues, disease develops.

I recall a beautiful woman in her mid-thirties who had been "constipated since I was a child." Besides feeling tired and lacking in the energy she believed she should have for a woman her age, she also had complained for many years of abdominal tenderness. After a series of colon irrigations the abdominal tenderness disappeared, and her energy level far exceeds her expectations.

The one matter for concern with the colon irrigation is that it needs to be done by qualified people using proper equipment. Any flora lost during the therapy needs to be replaced and instruments must be properly sterilized. It may seem as though the irrigation is hardly natural, but then, neither is an overburdened colon.

Color Therapy

This form of therapy has been receiving considerable attention over the past few years. It was used by the ancient Chinese who used to wrap people who had smallpox in a red cloth. Color seems to affect the mood and health of the body. It can also be used to heal. The "frequency" of the color — the rate that it pulses — is what heals. It is picked up by nerve endings in the skin called dermatones.

Blue and green light produce a calming, soothing, cooling effect. These colors are useful in treating an inflammation. Oranges, reds and yellows, on the other hand, are stimulating to the body and are useful in increasing circulation.

Colored lights are often used in conjunction with other healing techniques. For example, a cold-water pack may be applied to an inflamed area. Following this, the area may be placed under a blue or green light. If an area has been hurt by a fall, blood will rush to the injured area. If the area is covered with a cool compress and then later placed under a green light, a soothing effect will occur.

Cranial Moulding

The skull actually comprises many smaller bones that, as we grow, join along suture lines. Because of trauma in childhood or even later in life, sutures can be misaligned. These misalignments can result in conditions such as chronic sinus problems, or even migraine headaches. Through gentle manipulation of the sutures, the skull can be re-aligned, resulting in many beneficial effects.

Fever Therapy

This therapy has its roots in Germany. A patient was placed into a hot chamber and the temperature was gradually increased until a fever was produced. The object was to destroy old conditions locked in the body and draw them out through the skin. (The natural healer always draws old conditions out from the body, while the allopathic physician with his salves and ointments drives them further in.) Often as patients undergo fever therapy, they re-experience feelings and thoughts they had at the time the old condition was affecting them.

Footbaths

Originating in Germany, footbaths are another cleansing therapy. They use the principle of osmosis to remove toxins from the bloodstream. Osmosis is the tendency of fluids separated by a porous partition to pass through it and mix with each other. If the density and pressure of one fluid is lower, then it will pass into the fluid of higher density and pressure. The solution into which the foot is placed in a footbath has a greater density than that within the body. Thus it draws toxins, uric acid, and mucous out through the skin and into the water. Because our blood is constantly circulating, not only corpuscles in the feet are cleansed, but also those in other parts of the body for their source of blood is the circulating bloodstream. Because the skin is a semipermeable membrane, it allows fluids to pass through it. We are, of course, all familiar with perspiration, which the body eliminates.

This treatment is usually a pleasant one for patients. They take twenty minutes out of their busy days to sit and relax and soak their feet in a therapeutic bath of britannical herbs.

Immersion Bath

The body's third largest waste disposal unit — after the bowels and lungs — is the skin. By immersing the body in warm water to which specific herbs have been added, many effects can be produced. The body can be calmed, skin irritations can be soothed, and waste products can be drawn out.

Inhalation Therapy

This therapy brings herbs in the form of a vapor to sinuses and bronchi. This procedure is performed in a doctor's office as a compressor and inhalation mask must be used. Essential britannicals are put in liquid form. Cool air is blown past them to form a vapor. This is breathed in and affects either the sinuses or bronchi depending upon the need. On occasion other herbs are useful for relieving headaches.

Massage

This is perhaps one of the oldest forms of healing, although over the past ten years it has enjoyed a rejuvenation. For generations mothers have stroked their ill children to comfort, ease, and relax the child. Massage benefits the circulatory and lymphatic systems. It also has a way of releasing stress from the musculo-skeletal system. The motion of the hands of the therapist determine whether there will be a calming or a stimulating response in the body. Massage is very helpful in rehabilitating the musculo-skeletal system following traumatic injury.

Music Therapy

Music can be extremely soothing. It is now being used even on dairy and chicken farms as a tool for increased productivity. Cows produce more milk and chickens produce more eggs when they listen to music. Some offices play music for their employees. This subject will certainly be investigated more over the next twenty years. Suffice it to say that a room lit in blues and greens in which soothing music is being played would benefit any harried city-dweller at the end of a day.

Osteopathic Manipulation

This type of healing has its roots in ancient Egypt. The bony form of the body is manipulated and used as a lever to promote proper circulation, which is essential for health. Though osteopathy resembles chiropractic in its manipulations, its object is to increase circulation, whereas chiropractic works with the nervous system. In actuality, the two therapies are very different from each other.

Poultices

Poultices have been used for hundreds of years to cleanse the body and reduce inflammation. Clay poultices are used a great deal to drain impurities from the liver. Castor oil poultices help drain the gall bladder. Hayseed or comfrey poultices will relieve inflammation. A cabbage and carrot poultice can relieve a sore throat. A hot potato poultice will relieve an earache.

Reflexology

The feet represent a map of the body. Sensitivities on various points of the foot are an indication of weaknesses or illnesses. The sensitive areas are caused by a build up of uric acid crystals. When pressure is applied to the affected area, the crystals are disbursed.

Shiatsu

Shiatsu is the Japanese form of acupuncture. It is done by applying pressure with the fingers to various points of the body and head in order to balance the meridians and create a better flow of energy through the body. It has a calming yet stimulating effect on both body and mind.

Structural Alignment

This healing therapy developed by Ida Rolf in the early part of this century is based on the idea that there should be a balance between the body and gravity. If there is a balance, then stresses and strains to the body will not take place. The Rolfer's work is to balance the musculo-skeletal structure and the body's frame so that the new position allows the body to avoid faulty pulls against gravity. If we dropped a plumb bob from the ear, it should follow a straight line through the shoulder, hip, leg and ankle. That is the Rolfer's goal.

BIBLIOGRAPHY

Abrahamson, E.M. and A.W. Pezet. *Body, Mind and Sugar.* New York: Holt, Rinehart and Winston, 1965.

Aird, Bentall and Fraser Roberts. *British Journal Of Medicine.* April, 1953, 799 – 801.

Amend, Eleanor E. *A Synopsis of Natural Healing Methods.* Phoenix: Brehm Enterprises, n.d.

Anderson, Mary. *Colour Healing.* Wallingburgh, U.K.: Thorson's Publishers Ltd., 1975.

Ardell, Donald B. *High Level Wellness.* Emmaus, Pa.: Rodale Press, 1977.

Ash, Dr. Michael. *The Handbook of Natural Healing.* Cornwall, U.K.: Camspress, 1977.

Atkins, Robert C. and Shirley Linde. *Dr. Atkins' Superenergy Diet.* New York: Crown Publishers Inc., 1977.

Bailey, Herbert. *The Vitamin Pioneers.* New York: Pyramid Books, 1970.

——*Vitamin E Your Key to a Healthy Heart.* New York: Arc Books, 1966.

Banik, Dr. Allen E. and Reneé Taylor. *Hunza Land.* Long Beach, Calif.: Whitehorn Publishing Co., 1960.

Beesley, R.P. *The Robe of Many Colours.* Sussex, U.K.: Whitelodge Publications, 1974.

Berland, Theodore and editors of *Consumers Guide. Rating the Diets.* Consumers Guide, 1974.

Bieler, Henry G. *Food is Your Best Medicine.* New York: Vintage, Random House, 1973.

Bricklin, Mark, ed. *The Practical Encyclopedia of Natural Healing.* Emmaus, Pa.: Rodale Press Inc., 1976.

Buchanan and Higley. *British Journal of Exp. Pathology.* 1921, 2:227.

Buckwalter. *Journal of the American Medical Association.* Vol. 103, No. 13, 1956, pp. 1215 – 1217.

Carey, Dr. George W. *The Chemistry and Wonders of the Human Body.* Los Angeles, Chemistry of Life Co., 1963.

Church, Walter ed. *A Garland of Wisdom.* Virginia Beach: A.R.E. Press, 1975.

D'Adamo, Dr. James with Alan Richards. *One Man's Food.* New York: Richard Merek Publishers, 1980.

Dilfer, Carol Stahmann. *Your Baby, Your Body.* New York: Crown Publishers Inc., 1977.

Ewald, Ellen Buchman. *Recipes for a Small Planet.* New York: Ballantine Books, 1973.

Gabel, Medard. *Ho-Ping: Food for Everyone.* New York: Anchor Press / Doubleday, 1979.

Grossinger, Richard. *Planet Medicine,* revised edition. Boulder, Colorado: Shambala Publications Inc., 1982.

Hawkins, David and Linus Pauling eds. *Orthomolecular Psychiatry.* San Francisco, W.W. Freeman and Co., 1973.

Hunt, Roland. *Fragrant and Radiant Healing Symphony.* 1949.

Kellogg, J.H. *The Itinerary of a Breakfast.* New York: Funk and Wagnalls Co., 1926.

Kent, James Tyler. *Lectures on Homeopathic Philosophy.* New Delhi, B. Jain Publishers, 1970.

Kervan, Louis C. trans. Michel Abehsera. *Biological Transmutations.* Binghamton, New York: Swan House Publishing Co., 1972.

Kirschmann, John D. *Nutrition Almanac.* New York: McGraw-Hill Book Co., 1975.

Kriege, Theodor. trans. A.W. Priest. *Fundamental Basis of Iris Diagnosis.* London: L.N. Fowler and Co. Ltd., 1975.

Langman, *Gut.* 1965, 6:270.

Lappe, Frances Moore and Joseph Collins with Cary Fowler. *Food First.* New York: Ballantine Books, 1978.

Lawson-Wood, D. and J. *Glowing Health.* Rushington, Sussex: Health Science Press, 1961.

Lilliston, Lynn. *Megavitamins: A New Key to Health.* Greenwich, Conn.: Fawcett Publications Inc., 1975.

Lovell, Dr. Philip M. *Arthritis.* Costa Mesa, Calif.: Natural Health Publications, 1964.

——*Nervous Tension.* Costa Mesa, Calif.: Natural Health Publications, 1964.

Manner, Harold W., Steven J. Di Santi and Thomas L. Michalsen. *The Death of Cancer.* Chicago, Advanced Century Publishing Corp., 1978.

Mellan, Ibert and Eleanor. *Poisons.* New York: Pyramid Books, 1962.

Merikas. *American Journal of Digestive Diseases.* 10, 1966, pp. 11 – 16.

Mindell, Earl. *Earl Mindell's Vitamin Bible.* New York: Warner Books, 1979.

Newton, Marceline A. *The New Life Cookbook.* Norfolk, Virginia: Donning, 1976.

Norris, P.E. *About Nuts and Dried Fruit.* London: Thorson's Publishers Ltd., 1966.

Obannon, Kathleen. *Energy Health and Beauty.* Toronto: Natural Light Publishing Co., 1979.

Orton, James and Otto Newhaus. *Human Biochemistry.* 9th edition. St. Louis: C.V. Mosby, 1979.

Pearson, Durk and Sandy Shaw. *Life Extension.* New York: Warner Books, 1982.

Robertson, Laurel, Carol Flinders and Bronwen Godfrey. *Laurel's Kitchen.* Berkeley: Nilgiri Press, 1976.

Rosenberg, Dr. Harold and A.N. Feldzman. *The Doctor's Book of Vitamin Therapy.* New York: G.P. Putnam's Sons, 1974.

Rosner, Fred and Suessman Munter, trans. and ed. *The Medical Aphorisms of Moses Maimonedes.* Vol. I and II. New York: Bloch Publishing Co., 1973.

Shelton, Herbert M. *Health for Millions.* Chicago: Natural Hygiene Press Inc., 1968.

Stephan, Peter M. *The Secret of Eternal Youth.* New York: Arco Publishing Co. Inc., 1971.

Thomson, James C., *Sleep for the Sleepless*. Edinburgh: T.K. Publications, n.d.

Twelve Steps and Twelve Traditions. New York: Alcoholics Anonymous Publishing, 1973.

Ugelli, L. *Policlinico*. Sez Prat, 1936, 43:1591.

Verner, J.R., C.W. Weiant and R.J. Watkins. *Rational Bacteriology*. second edition. New York: H. Wolff, 1953.

Verny, Thomas with John Kelly. *The Secret Life of the Unborn Child*. New York: Delta, Dell Publishing Co. Inc., 1981.

Von Haller, Albert. *The Vitamin Hunters*. New York: Chilton Co., 1962.

Watkins, Arthur L. *A Manual of Electrotherapy*. 2nd edition. Philadelphia: Lea and Fbiger, 1962.

Watson, Dr. George. *Nutrition and Your Mind*. New York: Bantam, Harper and Row, 1974.

Wendel, Dr. Paul. *Naturopathic Spinal Manipulative Technique*. Brooklyn, New York, n.p., n.d.

INDEX

Acne, 111, 115
    possible causes, and treatments,
    146
Acupuncture, 179
Additives, avoiding, 44
Air sickness, 113
Alcoholism, 116, 117
Allergies, 118
    possible causes, and treatments,
    154
Alzheimer's disease, 118
    possible causes, and treatments,
    147
Amygdalin, 117
Anemia, 115, 117, 124
    pernicious, 116
    possible causes, and treatments,
    147–48
    sickle-cell, 117
Angina, 121
Anorexia nervosa, possible causes,
    and treatments, 148
Antibodies, 118
Aromatherapy, 179

Arthritis, 115, 118, 124, 127
    possible causes, and treatments,
    148–49
Ascorbic acid. See Vitamin C
Asthma, 118, 120
    possible causes, and treatments,
    149
Atherosclerosis, 120
Atherosclerotic plaques, 115, 119

Baldness, 119
Beriberi, 113
Biotin, 118
Birth control pill, 115, 122
Blood, clotting, 122–23
Blood pressure (high), 122, 126
    possible causes, and treatments,
    149–50
Blood pressure (low), 123
    possible causes, and treatments,
    150
Blood types
    determining, 26–27
    different effects of, 14–16

Blood typing, 171, 173–74
Boils, 111
Bones, 121, 122, 126, 127
Bronchitis, possible causes, and
    treatments, 150–51
Burns, 121

Calcium, 122–23
Cancer, 117, 120
  possible causes, and treatments,
    151–52
Candida, 165
Caprylic acid, 165
Carbuncles, 111
Carcinogens, 44
Cardiovascular system, 126
Cataracts, 113
Celiac disease, 122
Cells, 2–3
Chemicals, avoiding, 44
Children's diseases, 166–70
Chiropractic manipulation, 179–80
Chlorine, 123
Cholesterol, 115, 129
  in blood, 121–22, 123
Choline, 118
Chromium, 123
Circulatory problems, possible
    causes, and treatments, 152
Cleansing therapies, 177–86
Cobolamin (B$_{12}$), 116
Cobalt, 124
Coffee, avoiding, 43
Colds, 167
  in children, 167–68
Colitis, possible causes, and treat-
    ments, 153
Colon irrigation, 180–81
Color therapy, 182
Constipation, 116
  possible causes, and treatments,
    153–54
Cooking, do's and don'ts, 38–39
Copper, 124
Cranial moulding, 182
Cystitis, 165

DNA, 2–3, 116, 117
Dandruff, 127
Depression, 112, 113, 117, 123,
    124
Diabetes, 116, 121, 123
Diagnostic procedures, 171–75
Diarrhea, 114, 116, 117
Diuretic, 115, 126
Dizziness, 114, 126

Eating
  do's and don'ts, 39
  rules, 40
  what to avoid, 40–44
Eczema, 111, 119
  possible causes, and treatments,
    154
Eye conditions, possible causes,
    and treatments, 154–55
Eyes, 111

Family menus, 143–44
"Feeling full," 34–35
Fever
  in children, 167
  therapy, 182–83
Folic acid, 117
Food
  chemical structure of, 33
  combinations, significance of,
    34, 35–36
  habits, breaking, 11–13
Footbaths, 183
Funk, Casimir, 108

Gall bladder problems, possible
    causes, and treatments,
    155–56
Garlic, 165
Genetic weaknesses, strengthen-
    ing, 3
Goiter, 124
Gout, possible causes, and treat-
    ments, 156

Hair loss, 127
Hatha Yoga, 101, 105
Headaches, 114, 117, 124
Heart conditions, 121
  possible causes, and treatments,
    156–57
Heart disease, 116
Hemoglobin, 124
Hemorrhage, 121, 122
Herpes zoster, 113
High blood pressure, 122, 126,
  149–50
Hoffer, Abram, 114
Hyperactivity, 114
Hypertension, 128
Hypoglycemia, 41, 113
  possible causes, and treatments,
    157–58

Illness, attitudes to, 7–10
Immersion bath, 183
Immune system, 2, 127
Impetago, 111
Inhalation therapy, 183–84
Inner ear, 114
Inositol, 119
Insomnia, 114, 124
  possible causes, and treatments,
    159
Insulin, 41, 42
Insulin function, 123, 129
Iodine, 124
Iridology, 171–174
Iron, 124–25
Irritability, 112, 114, 117, 126

Junk food, increased consumption
  of, 44

Kidney, 127
Krohn's disease. *See* Colitis

Lactation, 113, 122
Laetrile, 117
Laxative, 120

Learning disorders, 114
Liver ailments, possible causes, and
  treatments, 159
Low back pain, possible causes,
  and treatments, 160
Low blood pressure, 123, 150
Lungs, 111
Lysine, 125

Magnesium, 125–26
Manganese, 126
Massage, 184
Memory, 126
Menopause, 122, 123, 128
Menstruation, 116, 165
Migraine, possible causes, and
  treatments, 160
Music therapy, 184

Naturopathic healing, 11
Nervous disorders, 115
Neuritis, possible causes, and treat-
  ments, 160–61
Niacin (B₃), 114–15
Nickel, 126
Night vision, 111

Osmond, Humphrey, 114
Osmotic pressure, 128
Osteopathic manipulation, 185
Osteoporosis, 123

PABA, 119
Pangamic acid (B₁₅), 116–17
Pantothenic acid, 118
Pauling, Linus, 108
Pellagra, 114
Pepsin, 34
Pesticides, in coffee, 43
Phosphorus, 126–27
Potassium, 127
Poultices, 185
Pregnancy, 111, 113, 117, 122
  morning sickness, 115
Prostate conditions, 129, 161

Psoriasis, possible causes, and
    treatments, 154
Psychosis, 117
Ptyalin, 34
Pulse diagnosis, 171, 174–75
Pyridoxine (B₆), 115–16

RNA, 116, 117
Recommended Dietary Allowances
    (RDA's), 109
Reflexology, 185
Responsibility for health, 5–7
Rheumatic diseases, 124
Rheumatoid arthritis, 113
Riboflavin (B₂), 113–14
Rickets, 121
Rolf, Ida, 186

Schizophrenia, 114, 124, 129
Scurvy, 120
Sedative, 119
Selenium, 127–28
Shiatsu, 186
Shopping, do's and don'ts, 37–38
Shute, Evan, 108, 121
Silicon, 129
Sinus conditions, 111, 120
    possible causes, and treatments,
        161–62
Skin rashes, 111, 115
Sodium, 128–29
Sore throats
    in children, 168–69
    possible causes, and treatments,
        161–62
Stomach, size of, 35
Stomach aches, 166
    in children, 170
Stress, 112, 120, 123, 126
Strokes, 128
Structural alignment, 186
Sugar, avoiding, 41–42
Sulphur, 128
Sunscreen, 119

T'ai Chi Ch'uan, 20, 105
Teeth, 122
Thiamine (B₁), 112–13
Thyroid, 124, 126
Tissues, 129
Tooth decay, 121
Tranquilizer, 119
Trichloroethylene, 43
Tryptophan, 129
Type A, 14, 15, 27
    child, 141–42
    making dietary changes by levels
        one, 96–97
        two, 97–98
        three, 98–99
        four, 99–100
        five, 100
    menus for, 54–59
    profile of, 18–21
    vitamin and mineral
        requirements, 132–33
Type AB, 15, 27
    child, 143
    making dietary changes by levels
        one, 104–105
        two, 105
        three, 105–106
        four, 106
        five, 107
    menus, for 66–69
    profile of, 23–25
    vitamin and mineral
        requirements, 133–34
    menus for, 81–84
    profile of, 30–31
    vitamin and mineral
        requirements, 136
Type Ao
    menus for, 77–80
    profile of, 30
    vitamin and mineral
        requirements, 135
Type B, 15, 27
    catarrhal nature, diet for, 102,
        103

child, 142
fatigued nature, diet for, 102, 103
making dietary changes by levels
one, 100
two, 101
three, 102–103
four, 103
five, 104
menus for, 60–65
profile of, 21–23
vitamin and mineral requirements, 133
Type Ba
menus for, 88–92
profile of, 32
vitamin and mineral requirements, 137
Type Bo
menus for, 84–88
profile of, 31–32
vitamin and mineral requirements, 136
Type O, 14, 15, 27
child, 140–41
making dietary changes by levels
one, 93–94
two, 94
three, 95
four, 95
five, 95–96
menus for, 46–53
profile of, 16–18
vitamin and mineral requirements, 131–32
Type Oa, 27
menus for, 69–73
profile of, 28–29
vitamin and mineral requirements, 134
Type Ob
menus for, 73–77
profile of, 29–30
vitamin and mineral requirements, 134–35

Ulcers, 115
possible causes, and treatments, 162
Urinary tract ailments, possible causes, and treatments, 162
Uterus, 111

Vaginal discharge (yeast), 165
Varicose veins, 121
possible causes, and treatments, 152–53
Vegetarian diet, suitability of, 15
Vitamin, origin of, 108
Vitamin A, 10–11
Vitamin B, 112
B$_1$, 112–13
B$_2$, 113–14
B$_3$, 114–15
B$_6$, 115–16
B$_{12}$, 116
B$_{15}$, 116–17
B$_{17}$, 117
Vitamin C, 119–20
Vitamin D, 121
Vitamin E, 121–22
Vitamin K, 122
Vitamins
healing capacity of, 108–109
as supplement to diet, 109–10

Wrinkles, 119

Yeast
and bloating, 163
getting rid of, 164–65
mental effects of, 174
vaginal, 165
Yoga, 20, 22, 23

Zinc, 129–30